Certified Coding Specialist– Physician-Based (CCS-P) Exam Preparation

Twelfth Edition

Anita C. Hazelwood, EdD, RHIA, FAHIMA

Lisa M. Delhomme, MHA, RHIA

Carol A. Venable, MPH, RHIA, FAHIMA

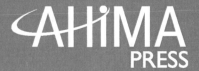
AHIMA PRESS

ISBN: 978-1-58426-861-1
eISBN: 978-1-58426-862-8

AHIMA Product No.: AC400222

AHIMA Staff:
Jessica Block, MA, Production Development Editor
Sarah Cybulski, MA, Assistant Editor
Megan Grennan, Director, Content Production and AHIMA Press
James Pinnick, Vice President, Content and Learning Solutions
Christine Scheid, Content Development Manager
Rachel Schratz, MA, Associate Digital Content Developer

Cover image: © 31moonlight31; iStock

For more information, including updates, about AHIMA Press publications, visit **http://www.ahima.org/education/press**.

American Health Information Management Association
233 North Michigan Avenue, 21st Floor
Chicago, Illinois 60601-5809
ahima.org

Contents

About the Contributing Editors

Anita C. Hazelwood, EdD, RHIA, FAHIMA, is a professor and the department head for Health Sciences in the College of Nursing and Health Sciences at the University of Louisiana at Lafayette. She has co-authored two AHIMA books titled *Diagnostic Coding for Physician Services: ICD-10* and *ICD-10-CM Preview*. Dr. Hazelwood was the recipient of the AHIMA Legacy Award and is a Fellow of the American Health Information Management Association.

Dr. Hazelwood has conducted numerous coding workshops at the local, state, and national levels. Moreover, she has published articles in *Educational Perspectives in Health Information Management* in addition to serving on its editorial review board.

Lisa M. Delhomme, MHA, RHIA, is the program director of the Health Information Management program at the University of Louisiana at Lafayette. She teaches courses in privacy and security, data analytics, and database management. Mrs. Delhomme is an active AHIMA volunteer and served on AHIMA's Council for Excellence in Education. She has served several volunteer roles with AHIMA and is a former President of the Louisiana Health Information Management Association. She is a frequent presenter at state and national conferences in her areas of expertise.

Carol A. Venable, MPH, RHIA, FAHIMA, is a retired professor and the former HIM department head from the University of Louisiana at Lafayette. Ms. Venable has co-authored two AHIMA books titled *Diagnostic Coding for Physician Services: ICD-10* and *ICD-10-CM Preview* and was a contributing author for the *Clinical Coding Workout* in 2011. She was the recipient of the AHIMA Legacy Award for one of the publications and is a Fellow of the American Health Information Management Association.

Ms. Venable has conducted numerous coding workshops at the local, state, and national levels. As an active volunteer for AHIMA and LHIMA, she has served on numerous committees.

Preface

The twelfth edition of *CCS-P Exam Preparation* is designed to help you study for the certified coding specialist–physician-based (CCS-P) exam. To become a physician-based coding professional, you need proficiency in assigning numeric codes for each diagnosis and procedure, in-depth knowledge of the Current Procedural Terminology (CPT) coding system, and familiarity with the *International Classification of Diseases, Tenth Revision, Clinical Modification* (ICD-10-CM) and Healthcare Common Procedure Coding System (HCPCS) Level II coding systems. This exam preparation guide will help you prepare for the CCS-P certification exam and help you identify less competent areas for further study. However, if at this point in your endeavor your knowledge in any area is not as solid as it should be, we highly recommend you obtain the following AHIMA publication for study:

> *Procedural Coding and Reimbursement for Physician Services: Applying Current Procedural Terminology and HCPCS*, 2021, by Kim Huey, MJ, CCS-P, CHC, COC, CPC, CPCO, PCS

Other AHIMA publications cover topics such as health information documentation, data integrity and quality, and additional key areas of expertise required by the coding professional in the physician practice (available at AHIMA's webstore, https://my.ahima.org/store/).

To fully prepare for the CCS-P exam, consult AHIMA's certification website (https://www .ahima.org/certification-careers/certification-exams/) to check eligibility requirements, download and submit an exam application, see sample test questions and screenshots of the exam format, view a list of study resources, and find out more about exam day procedures, including which code books are allowed.

The CCS-P exam assesses mastery-level knowledge and proficiency in coding rather than entry-level skills. The certification exam is based on an explicit set of competencies that have been determined by job analysis surveys of coding professionals in physician-based practices. Those competencies are subdivided into domains and tasks that include health information documentation, ICD-10-CM diagnosis coding, CPT and HCPCS Level II coding, as well as reimbursement, data quality and analysis, information and communication technologies, and compliance and regulatory issues. Thorough preparation to take the CCS-P exam suggests that you have already successfully encountered and mastered questions in each of these domains. The practice medical scenario questions require diagnostic (ICD-10-CM) coding in all specialties and procedural (CPT and HCPCS Level II) coding for physician services.

Clearly, the best preparation for the exam is your education. We offer this exam preparation guide to help you succeed on the CCS-P exam. The editors have used their collective expertise to compile questions that are aligned to the content areas currently featured on the exam. The variety of questions ensures you have experience with all approaches.

Congratulations! You have chosen to earn a credential in a rewarding professional field.

About the CCS-P Exam

The CCS-P credential-holder is a coding practitioner with expertise in physician-based settings such as physician offices, group practices, multispecialty clinics, or specialty centers. This coding practitioner reviews patients' records and assigns numeric codes for each diagnosis and procedure. To perform this task, an individual must possess in-depth knowledge of the CPT coding system and familiarity with the ICD-10-CM and HCPCS Level II coding systems. The CCS-P is also an expert in health information documentation, data integrity, and quality. Because patients' coded data are submitted to insurance companies or the government for expense reimbursement, the CCS-P plays a crucial role in the health provider's business operation.

The CCS-P certification exam assesses mastery or proficiency in coding rather than entry-level skills. If you perform coding in a physician's office, clinic, or similar setting, consider obtaining the CCS-P certification to attest to your ability.

To help you study for the certification exam, *CCS-P Exam Preparation* provides four practice exams that each include eight medical records from the hospital, emergency room, operating room, and physician's office or clinic settings for medical coding fill-in-the-blank practice. In addition, each of these exams includes 97 single-response multiple choice questions.

Detailed information about the CCS-P exam and academic eligibility requirements can be found at https://www.ahima.org/certification-careers/certification-exams/ccs-p/.

Exam Competency Statements

The CCS-P certification exam is based on an explicit set of competencies. These competencies were determined by job analysis surveys of physician-based coding professionals. The competencies are subdivided into domains and tasks as listed here.

Domain 1: Diagnosis Coding

Domain 2: Procedure Coding

Domain 3: Research

Domain 4: Compliance

Domain 5: Revenue Cycle

A full description of the tasks and exam specifications, as well as other exam preparation materials, including the list of allowable code books, can be found at https://www.ahima.org/certification -careers/certification-exams/ccs-p/.

A Note on *CCS-P Exam Preparation* Medical Scenarios

There are slight differences between the medical scenarios presented in this preparation guide and the medical scenarios on the CCS-P exam. On the exam, the test-taker will be asked to reference code books to select codes from a list provided under each category. The book has answer blanks for each code and does not provide a preselected list of codes from which to choose. The book intentionally provides these answer blanks to create a more challenging self-testing environment for the user.

This book presents medical scenarios for coding as a component, and the answers are grouped into three categories: principal diagnosis, additional diagnosis codes, and procedure codes. The sequencing of codes within the categories is not tested on the online assessment that accompanies this book.

CCS-P Exam Preparation contains four complete practice exams with 8 medical scenarios each and an additional 20 practice scenarios, for a total of 52 medical scenarios. The documentation-based coding scenarios are one of the most valuable aspects of the materials presented in the book and corresponding online assessment.

Completing the scenarios in this guide will provide prospective test-takers with practice in real-world coding they may be required to complete as a working physician-based coding professional when they will need to assign a code chosen from a code book or encoder. By requiring a more rigorous and variable coding process of the user, the medical scenarios in *CCS-P Exam Preparation* will prepare examinees for coding health records on the examination and beyond.

Procedures for Coding the Medical Scenarios in This Book

- Apply ICD-10-CM instructional notations and conventions and current approved Diagnostic Coding and Reporting Guidelines for Outpatient Services (Section IV of the official *ICD-10-CM Guidelines for Coding and Reporting*), to select diagnoses, conditions, problems, or other reasons for care that require ICD-10-CM coding in a physician-based encounter either in a physician's office, clinic, outpatient area, emergency room, ambulatory surgery, or other ambulatory care setting. Code for professional services only.
- Sequencing is not required for the diagnoses or procedures.
- Apply the following directions to assign codes to secondary diagnoses:
  - Chronic diseases treated on an ongoing basis may be coded and reported as many times as the patient is receiving treatment and care for the condition(s).
  - Code all documented conditions that coexist at the time of the encounter and that require or affect patient care, treatment, or management.
  - Conditions previously treated and no longer existing are not coded.
- Code for the professional services only and only for the physician or surgeon designated in each individual medical scenario.
- Assign two-character HCPCS Level II codes for all appropriate services.
- Assign CPT codes for anesthetic procedures listed in the anesthesia section only if indicated on the medical scenario cover sheet.
- Assign CPT codes for medical services and procedures based on current CPT guidelines.
- Confirm evaluation and management (E/M) codes based on the information provided in the box for each medical scenario.
  For the purposes of this examination, do not challenge the level of key components chosen. You will not be expected to assign the level of history, examinations, and medical decision-making.
- Assign CPT codes for radiology and pathology/laboratory procedures listed in the radiology and pathology/laboratory sections only when applicable.
- Assign CPT codes from the medicine section based on current CPT guidelines.
- Assign five-digit HCPCS Level II (alphanumeric) codes, as appropriate.
- Do not assign ICD-10-CM External Causes of Morbidity codes (V00–V99, Chapter 20).
- Assign ICD-10-CM Factors Influencing Health Status and Contact with Health Services codes (Z00–Z99, Chapter 21) as appropriate.
- Do not assign ICD-10-PCS codes.
- Do not assign Category II or Category III CPT codes.

For the most up-to-date exam information, visit https://www.ahima.org/certification-careers/certification-exams/.

How to Use This Book

The CCS-P practice questions and practice exams in this guide and with the accompanying online assessments test knowledge of content pertaining to the CCS-P domains. This book contains four complete practice exams, each made up of 97 single-response multiple choice questions and 8 medical scenarios. Each multiple-choice question is identified by a CCS-P domain, so you will be able to determine whether you need knowledge or skill building in particular areas of the exam competencies. All answers include a rationale and corresponding reference. Pursuing these references will help you build your knowledge and skills in specific domains.

The most effective way to use this guide is to work through each practice exam in the allotted exam time. You will find information about the allotted exam time at https://www.ahima.org /certification-careers/certification-exams/ccs-p/. Identify areas in which you may need further preparation. For any questions you answer incorrectly, read the associated references to refresh your knowledge.

About the Online Assessments

The self-scoring practice questions can be set to be presented in random order, or you may choose to go through the questions in sequential order by domain. You may also choose to practice or test your skills on specific domains. For example, if you would like to build your coding skills in domains 1 and 2, you may choose only those domains' multiple choice and multiple select questions for a given practice session.

Acknowledgments

The editors and AHIMA Press would like to thank Roger Hettinger, MBA, RHIA, CCS, CCS-P, CHTS-IS, COC, CPC, CRCR, and Cari Greenwood, RHIA, CCS, CICA, CPC, for their technical review of this edition.

Introduction

This publication is designed to help you prepare for the AHIMA certified coding specialist–physician-based (CCS-P) examination. There are four practice exams, which include practice questions and medical scenarios.

Included in this introduction are 20 medical scenarios for immediate practice.

After working through the practice exams and medical scenarios in the book, candidates should test their knowledge of the material contained in the domains covered by the exam.

Introductory Medical Scenarios

PRACTICE—SCENARIO 1

PROCEDURE NOTE:

FINDINGS: There was a 1.6 × 1.5-cm congenital defect of the right nasal sidewall that did not involve the alar cartilages. It did extend slightly onto the cheek.

PROCEDURE: After obtaining informed consent, the patient was taken into the operating room and placed in a supine position on the operating table. General anesthesia was induced via endotracheal intubation without difficulty. Approximately 2 mL of 1% lidocaine with 1:100,000 epinephrine was injected into the right conchal bowl and the right postauricular region. The face was prepped and draped in a sterile fashion. A surgical pause was performed to confirm the patient's identity and site of surgery.

A skin incision was made in the conchal bowl on the right-hand side, and a piece of conchal bowl cartilage measuring approximately 1 × 1.5 cm was harvested and placed in saline to be used as a strut along the right lateral sidewall. This incision was closed using 6-0 fast-absorbing gut.

A piece of foil was used to create a template of the defect in the nose. A full-thickness skin graft matching to the shape of a template was harvested from the right postauricular region. The cartilage was then placed along the lateral sidewall and secured in place with a single through-and-through fast-absorbing gut suture. The central portion of the full-thickness skin graft was also secured with a fast-absorbing gut suture to the central portion of the nasal defect. The perimeter of the graft was then sutured to the nose using interrupted 6-0 nylon suture.

Once the graft had been sutured in place, the harvested site in the postauricular region was expanded into an elliptical-shaped defect by removing some skin superior and inferior to the harvest site itself. Undermining was performed primarily in the posterior direction of the skin under the hairline. Minimal undermining was done of the skin anteriorly toward the pinna of the ear. Hemostasis was obtained after the undermining, and this harvest site incision was closed using 4-0 Vicryl and 5-0 nylon. A small pressure dressing was applied to the right side of the nose, and a Glasscock mastoid dressing was placed on the right ear.

The patient was then awakened from the anesthetic, extubated, and transported to the recovery room with stable vital signs and no evidence of stridor.

Enter one diagnosis code and two procedure codes.

DX1 [ ]

PR1 [ ]

PR2 [ ]

PRACTICE—SCENARIO 2

PREOPERATIVE DIAGNOSIS: Nontraumatic right hip labral tear

POSTOPERATIVE DIAGNOSIS: Nontraumatic right hip labral tear

ANESTHESIA: General endotracheal

PROCEDURE: Right hip arthroscopic labral debridement

COMPLICATIONS: None

DRAINS: None

ESTIMATED BLOOD LOSS: Minimal

PROPHYLAXIS: Ancef

OPERATIVE FINDINGS: The patient was noted to have a labral tear in the superior portion of the acetabular labrum with a frayed portion of the labrum hanging down inferiorly. Patient was also noted to have some tearing of the tissue along the pulvinar at the attachment of the ligamentum along the acetabular side as well. No articular lesions seen. No loose bodies seen. No other significant findings.

INDICATION FOR PROCEDURE: The patient is a 22-year-old female complaining of right hip pain. MRI confirms evidence of a labral tear. The patient also had a diagnostic injection with relief of pain and requires a right hip arthroscopic labral debridement versus repair. I discussed with the patient all risks, benefits, alternatives, and complications of the procedure including, but not limited to, infection, bleeding, damage to nerves or blood vessels, failure to relieve hip pain, decreased range of motion, reaction to anesthesia, etc. She understands and would like to proceed with operative intervention.
All questions were answered. Consent is signed and on the chart prior to the start of the procedure.

PROCEDURE IN DETAIL: After the patient indicated that the right hip was the correct operative site, it was marked in the pre-op holding area by the surgeon. The patient was then taken to the operating room and placed in the supine position on the Chick table with all bony prominences adequately padded. Perineal post was placed.
A Foley catheter was placed. The patient was placed in boots bilaterally, and traction was applied with the patient's hip in slight abduction and neutral rotation. Fluoroscopic images done by Radiology demonstrated an appropriate distraction. Traction was then let off. The right hip and lower extremity were then prepped and draped in the normal sterile fashion. Traction was applied, and time out was called in the room prior to incision. Next using fluoroscopic guidance, a spinal needle was passed at the anterolateral portal staying just anterior to the greater trochanter approximately 2 cm. Spinal needle was easily advanced into the hip joint. Hip articulation with an air arthrogram was achieved under fluoroscopy. Next, Nitinol wire was passed through this needle into the hip joint and after making an incision with a #11 blade and having infiltrated the joint with saline with good return, a trocar was then advanced into the hip articulation with a 5.5 cannula placed. Arthroscope was then placed, and diagnostic arthroscopy was performed with the abovementioned findings. Next, at the intersection of the greater trochanter and anterior superior iliac spine at the anterior portal needle localization under direct visualization was done, noting good placement within the hip joint. Through a percutaneous incision once again, another 5.5 cannula was placed, and a soft tissue shaver and electrocautery were then used to debride the frayed tissue at the pulvinar, as well as address the superior labral tear. This was probed and noted to have a flap tear particularly on the undersurface. Using both the flexible probe cautery as well as a curve and straight meniscal shaver through these cannulas by alternating between the anterolateral and anterior portals visualization as well as addressing this labral tear with debridement was accomplished successfully, debriding the labrum back to a stable rim. Remaining labrum was then probed and noted to be stable. The debridement was carried down onto the bone just on the undersurface of the labrum without injuring articular cartilage to allow for healing. Final arthroscopic images were obtained. After removal of these cannulas, traction was let down and portal sites were closed with 3-0 Vicryl subcutaneous sutures followed by Steri-Strips. Sterile dressing was applied. The patient was extubated in the operating room and transported to the recovery room without complication. All needle, sponge, and instrument counts were correct.

Enter one diagnosis code and one procedure code.

DX1

PR1

PRACTICE—SCENARIO 3

MR #: 353901

ENDOSCOPY REPORT

PREOPERATIVE DIAGNOSIS: Generalized abdominal pain

POSTOPERATIVE DIAGNOSIS: Grossly normal colonoscopy

RELEVANT HISTORY AND PHYSICAL FINDINGS: Abdominal pain for years, much improved recently on Activia

MEDICATIONS: None

DIET MODIFICATIONS: Daily Activia

The procedures were explained to the patient, including the purpose, risks, and benefits, and possible alternative procedures were discussed. Consent was obtained. The planned procedures were confirmed with staff, and the patient's identity was confirmed.

The patient was placed under general anesthesia with ET by an anesthesiologist. Photos were taken throughout the procedure. The PCF 160AL was passed via anus. The anus was normally placed. No fissures were observed. No fistulas were observed. No skin tags, no hemorrhoids or rash. The scope was passed. The preparation of the colon at this point was good. The anatomy of the rectum was normal. The mucosa was normal in color and vascularity. Biopsies were taken. The sigmoid anatomy was normal. The mucosa was normal in color and vascularity. Biopsies were taken. Transcending and ascending were both normal appearing. Biopsies taken in the transverse. The cecum was normal. The ICV was visualized and was normal. The terminal ileum was entered. It appeared normal.

COMPLICATIONS: None

The patient was repositioned. The GIF 140 was placed in the mouth and advanced through the mouth and hypopharynx under direct vision. The hypopharynx and cords were normal. Mucosa in the body of the esophagus was normal. The diaphragmatic indentation was visible. The Z line was identified. Biopsies were taken.

The scope was advanced into the stomach, which was insufflated with air. The anatomy was normal. Mucosa of the body, antrum, and pylorus were normal. Biopsies were taken of the antrum and body.

A turnaround procedure was performed. The gastroesophageal junction was normal. Biopsies were taken in the cardia.

The endoscope was advanced to the third portion of the duodenum. The ampulla of Vater was observed. The duodenal folds were normal. The mucosa was normal and velvety. Biopsies × 4 were taken in standard fashion with minimal traction of the duodenal mucosa away from the muscular wall. The jejunum was normal. The endoscope was withdrawn into the stomach, which was evacuated of air. The endoscope was removed.

COMPLICATIONS: None

RESULTS: Grossly normal colonoscopy and upper endoscopy

DISPOSITION: The patient was informed of the gross results of the exam. Biopsy results will be reported when received.

Enter one diagnosis code and two procedure codes.

DX1

PR1

PR2

PRACTICE—SCENARIO 4

PREOPERATIVE DIAGNOSIS: Acute respiratory failure, intracranial hemorrhage

POSTOPERATIVE DIAGNOSIS: Acute respiratory failure, intracranial hemorrhage

PROCEDURE PERFORMED: Tracheostomy

ANESTHESIA TYPE: General

ESTIMATED BLOOD LOSS: 10 mL

HISTORY: This is a 58-year-old female who presented with acute respiratory failure and intracranial hemorrhage. She has been on the ventilator and unable to support her ventilation without a mechanical ventilator. She is unable to be weaned from a ventilator and thus in need of a tracheostomy. The risks and benefits were explained to the family, and they consented to the procedure.

PROCEDURE: The patient was brought to the operating room and had preoperative antibiotics given prior to any incision. She had come down with the ET-tube, and this was hooked up to the ventilator by the anesthesia staff. She was prepped and draped in normal sterile fashion, and the anatomic landmarks of the thyroid cartilage and sternal notch were identified, as well as the cricothyroid membrane. About 1 fingerbreadth below the cricothyroid membrane, incision was made down to the level of the subcutaneous tissue. Bovie electrocautery was used to dissect down through the platysma. Any venous bleeders were identified and tied off with silk suture. We then had good exposure of the trachea. We identified the third tracheal ring. We had the ICU staff deflate the balloon and we placed stay sutures laterally on both sides of the third tracheal ring. This was carried down from skin to the tracheal ring back up to the skin. We then reinflated the balloon and then when we were ready we deflated the balloon again and made a square incision around the third tracheal ring and removed this portion in a square fashion. We brought our ET-tube out just proximal to this and used a tracheal spreader to dilate the trachea. We then placed a #8 Shiley tracheostomy tube without any difficulty, and the balloon was inflated. We then hooked our tracheostomy to the ventilator and received good end tidal CO_2. The patient was oxygenating at 100%, and her tidal volumes were equivalent to what they were pre-op with the ET-tube. There were no signs of bleeding, and good hemostasis was achieved. The skin around the tracheostomy incision was closed in running fashion, and the tracheostomy was secured in four places with nylon suture. The Vicryl stay sutures were secured to the chest wall with Steri-Strips. The patient tolerated the procedure well and was taken to ICU in stable condition.

Enter two diagnosis codes and one procedure code.

DX1

DX2

PR1

PRACTICE—SCENARIO 5

PREOPERATIVE DIAGNOSIS: Carcinoma of the right breast, status post neoadjuvant chemotherapy

POSTOPERATIVE DIAGNOSIS: Carcinoma of the right breast, status post neoadjuvant chemotherapy

PROCEDURE PERFORMED: Right modified radical mastectomy, subsequent reconstruction

PREOPERATIVE HISTORY: The patient is a 37-year-old female who had a pregnancy-associated breast cancer of the right breast with extensive involvement of the breast, clinically a stage III breast cancer. She underwent neoadjuvant chemotherapy with a complete clinical response to therapy with no residual palpable tumor in the breast and no palpable adenopathy. She has elected to undergo a right modified radical mastectomy with reconstruction, and we are taking her to the operating room now.

OPERATIVE NOTE: The patient was taken to the operating room. General anesthesia was induced. A Foley catheter was inserted. Her arms were placed on pads. Her legs were placed on pads. Bear hugger was applied, and her entire upper torso was sterilely prepped and draped in usual fashion. Symmetric skin sparing mastectomy was planned, incorporating the nipple-areolar complex. An elliptical incision was created incorporating the nipple-areolar complex. Flaps were raised from the superior infraclavicular incision and a portion of the breast circumferentially to the midline and subsequently to the inframammary fold and subsequently out to the latissimus dorsi muscle. The breast was removed from the pectoralis major muscle incorporating the fascia, reflected laterally. The clavipectoral fascia was opened, and a level I and level II axillary lymph node dissection was performed, sparing the long thoracic and the thoracodorsal neurovascular bundle, as well as at least one intercostal brachial cutaneous nerve. There was no palpable adenopathy in level III. We dissected lymph nodes out from underneath the pectoralis major muscle and from underneath the brachial vessels. The axillary dissection was truncated at its lowest extent. The breast and axilla were marked for orientation, weighed, and sent to pathology. Irrigation was performed. Hemostasis was achieved where necessary using some Surgiclips and electrocautery. There was no evidence of bleeding at the end of the case. At this point, Dr. X took over for the reconstructive portion of the procedure. This completes our operative dictation.

Enter two diagnosis codes and one procedure code.

DX1

DX2

PR1

PRACTICE—SCENARIO 6

INPATIENT PULMONARY CONSULTATION:

The patient was seen and examined by the intensive care unit house staff. Please see their notes for further details. He is post-trauma day 7. Some of his injuries include right acetabulum fracture, right open talus, manubrium rib fracture, mediastinal hematoma, and pulmonary contusion.

This morning, the patient was initially a GCS of 7. We held his sedation. He did wake up and followed some intermittent commands. He is currently on morphine at 2 mg/hour and Ativan at 2 mg/hour.

His lungs are coarse bilaterally. He is on assist control, rate of 12, tidal volume 600, PEEP of 10, FiO2 of 0.4. His saturations have been greater than 96%. He persists in acute respiratory failure; however, his AA gradient has been improving and we will attempt to decrease his PEEP today. Patient has a pulmonary contusion that I will continue to monitor.

CARDIOVASCULAR: His pulse is 80 to 115, blood pressure 100 to 130/60 to 80. He is in sinus tachycardia on examination.

RENAL/FLUID/ELECTROLYTES: He had 3.4 liters in and 2.4 liters out. His glucoses have been well controlled with EndoTool. His electrolytes are all within normal limits. His abdomen is much less distended than it has been over the previous several days. He is receiving tube feeds at 65 cc/hour.
He has had four bowel movements.

HEMATOLOGY: His hemoglobin is stable at 10. His platelet count is 225. He has on SCDs and is receiving Lovenox for DVT prophylaxis. T-max is 101.3. There is a much improved temperature curve and his white blood cell count is down to 11 from 12. He is currently on Linezolid and tobramycin. His BAL from 09/09 grew out *Haemophilus influenzae* and now yeast. His urine and blood cultures from 09/12 are negative. We will start Diflucan today. We will also send stool for C-diff. We will await final cultures from BAL prior to discontinuing Linezolid. We will continue tobramycin for treatment of his *Haemophilus influenzae*.

I spent over 30 minutes at this patient's bedside assessing him and making critical care decisions.

ASSESSMENT:

1. *Haemophilus influenzae*

2. Candida of lung

Enter four diagnosis codes and one procedure code.

DX1

DX2

DX3

DX4

PR1

PRACTICE—SCENARIO 7

DATE OF BIRTH: 08/30/1949

ADMISSION DATE: 12/13/20XX

SURGERY DATE: 12/13/20XX

PREOPERATIVE DIAGNOSIS: Thyroid nodule

POSTOPERATIVE DIAGNOSIS: Necrotic thyroid nodule, Hashimoto's thyroiditis based on frozen section

PROCEDURE: Right thyroid lobectomy and frozen section

ESTIMATED BLOOD LOSS: 30 mL

With adequate sedation in the operating room, the patient was given a general anesthetic. The patient was positioned and prepared and draped for thyroidectomy. A collar incision was performed after the skin was appropriately marked for symmetry. The skin, subcutaneous tissue, and platysmal muscle were divided, and then superior-inferior flaps were developed behind the platysmal muscle. The strap muscles were separated in the midline. There was a dominant nodule in the right lobe of the thyroid. The left lobe appeared grossly normal, although slightly enlarged and fleshy. Previous imaging had demonstrated some cystic change in the left lobe as well, but this was not apparent on gross examination. The right thyroid lobe was mobilized first by double ligating the superior thyroid vessels and then transected, and the thyroid gland mobilized. The parathyroid glands were not definitely visualized, but care was taken to dissect exactly on the capsule of the thyroid lobe. The recurrent laryngeal nerve was carefully identified and preserved. The inferior thyroidal vessels were clamped, transected, and ligated. Other bleeders were identified and secured with ligatures of 3-0 silk as well. The isthmus was transected and transfixed with two transfixion stitches of 3-0 silk. Hemostasis was then satisfactory. Frozen section revealed a mass with a necrotic center and a thin wall, which showed no malignant change. Permanent sections pending. The strap muscles were then approximated in the midline with a running simple stitch of 3-0 Vicryl. The platysmal muscle was approximated with interrupted simple stitches of 3-0 Vicryl and the skin was closed with 4-0 Vicryl. A sterile dressing was applied, and the patient left the operating room in satisfactory condition having tolerated the procedure satisfactorily.

Enter one diagnosis code and one procedure code.

DX1

PR1

PRACTICE—SCENARIO 8

PREOPERATIVE DIAGNOSIS: End-stage renal disease; Dialysis dependence

POSTOPERATIVE DIAGNOSIS: End-stage renal disease; Dialysis dependence

OPERATION: Left brachiocephalic arteriovenous fistula

ESTIMATED BLOOD LOSS: Less than 25 cc

COMPLICATIONS: None

PROCEDURE: The patient was taken to the operating room and placed in the supine position, where his left arm was placed on an arm board and prepared and draped in the usual sterile fashion. He was given intravenous sedation and a local anesthetic using 1% lidocaine. After infiltration of the area just above the antecubital fossa, an incision was made between the brachial artery and the cephalic vein and approximately 1 cm beyond the antecubital fossa proximally toward the shoulder. This was carried down through the skin and subcutaneous tissues to the level of the fascia. The fascia was identified, and dissection was continued laterally and medially to expose the cephalic vein, which was noted to have a medial branch that was large and clotted and a lateral branch that was a little smaller but clearly open. We traced the cephalic vein distally and proximally and developed enough mobility of the vein with ligation of branches and surrounding tissues to be able to move it toward the brachial artery for close approximation for anastomosis. Attention was then turned to the brachial artery, which was identified in a somewhat deep position in the medial aspect of the elbow and was noted to be relatively small with a diameter of around 4 to 5 mm. It had some mild disease in the arterial wall; however, after ligation of a single small branch, we were able to get elevation of approximately 2.5 cm of the artery. This provided adequate exposure for the arteriotomy and for proximal and distal occlusion. The patient then had amputation and ligation of the cephalic vein distally with the cut end being brought over to the artery. The artery itself was opened with a #11 blade after proximal and distal occlusion, and approximately 6 mm of anastomosis was performed in running fashion with 6-0 Prolene using the end of the spatulated cephalic vein to the side of the brachial artery. The patient tolerated this procedure very well. The anastomosis, once completed, did not bleed, and there was a good thrill in the vein. After inspection, there was no evidence of any significant obstruction to the vein course and no kinking that would cause any problems with development of the fistula.

At this point, we infiltrated the wounds with 0.25% Marcaine for postoperative anesthesia and closed the wounds with interrupted 3-0 Vicryl for the subcutaneous tissues and running 4-0 Monocryl for the skin. Sponge and needle counts were correct, and the patient was taken to recovery without incident with plan for discharge.

Enter two diagnosis codes and one procedure code.

DX1

DX2

PR1

PRACTICE—SCENARIO 9

DATE OF PROCEDURE: 03/07/20XX

HISTORY: This is a 59-year-old male with metastatic lung cancer who presented for EEG in the office with a diagnosis of status epilepticus on March 3, 20XX.

CONDITIONS: This is an 18-channel EEG done using the 10–20 system electrode placement. During the study, the patient was not able to follow commands and at times he groaned and yawned throughout this examination.

FINDINGS: The EEG begins with the patient's eyes closed and there is a posterior dominant rhythm of 7 on the left and 7 on the right. Photic stimulation and hyperventilation were not done. Sleep was not obtained. There was some left temporal slowing shown in leads T5-01 and FP1-F3. There was no epileptiform activity seen.

IMPRESSION: This is an abnormal EEG due to the slowing seen on the left temporofrontal area.

Enter one diagnosis code and one procedure code.

DX1

PR1

PRACTICE—SCENARIO 10

Please code for the services of the physician (professional) but do not assign a modifier.

REASON FOR EXAMINATION: Fourth nerve palsy

RESULTS:

CLINICAL HISTORY: Left fourth nerve palsy

EXAMINATION: MRI brain with and without contrast 1/18/20XX

COMPARISON: None

TECHNIQUE: Thin section axial T1, axial T2, T2, FLAIR, diffusion, ADC, and coronal T2, T1. Postcontrast T1 axial, thin section T1, sagittal, and coronal. 3 cc of gadolinium was used. Sedation was provided by anesthesia.

FINDINGS: No midline shift. No mass in the brain or brainstem. No abnormal signal in the brainstem. No abnormal signal or enhancement in the expected course of the fourth cranial nerves. Mild prominence of the supratentorial subarachnoid spaces. Third ventricle is mildly prominent. Lateral and fourth ventricles are normal. No mass or obstructing lesion in the aqueduct or tectum.

There are two ovoid, cystic foci in the periventricular white matter measuring 10 mm × 3 mm adjacent to the atria of the left lateral ventricle, likely prominent perivascular spaces.

No evidence of acute infarct on diffusion-weighted sequences.

No Chiari malformation. Normal corpus callosum. Normal myelination for age.

Paranasal sinuses and orbits are normal. There is diffuse high T2 signal in the mastoid air cells.

IMPRESSION:

1. Fourth cranial nerve palsy. No mass or abnormal signal in the brainstem. No abnormal signal or enhancement in the expected course of the fourth cranial nerves.

2. Mild prominence of the supratentorial subarachnoid spaces with mildly enlarged third ventricle and normal lateral and fourth ventricles. No obstructing mass identified, although communicating hydrocephalus could have this appearance.

Enter one diagnosis code and one procedure code.

DX1

PR1

PRACTICE—SCENARIO 11

ESTABLISHED PATIENT

HISTORY OF PRESENT ILLNESS: The patient is a 7-year-old boy who presents today with his mother due to jamming his finger in the door this morning. He caught his right middle finger in the door leading to his garage. It occurred about 40 minutes prior to his arrival at the clinic.

PHYSICAL EXAMINATION: Temperature 98.4, pulse 79, respirations 14, blood pressure 90/60. Heart has a regular rate and rhythm. Lungs are clear to auscultation. Abdomen is soft. The patient is alert and resting on his back on the examination table. An examination of the right middle finger shows some swelling and a flap of skin to the distal right middle finger that is raised. There appears to be no involvement of the nail bed itself, no subungual hematoma present. Distal extremity is neurovascularly intact.

RADIOGRAPHS: X-rays on the right middle finger done at the imaging center do not demonstrate any fracture to the distal tip. Await official report of radiology.

PROCEDURE: The patient was taken to the procedure room. Informed consent was obtained from the patient's mother, and she gave permission for laceration repair. He was placed in a supine position, and a digital block was performed with 2 mL of 2% lidocaine. The area was then cleansed and irrigated with copious amounts of sterile saline. The area was then draped in a sterile fashion and three 5-0 Ethilon interrupted sutures were placed to realign the 1-cm flap. Dressing was applied and patient tolerated it well.

ASSESSMENT: Laceration of the right middle finger

PLAN:

1. Status post repair.

2. Wound care directions were given. The patient will follow up in 7 to 10 days for suture removal or sooner if any condition worsens or problems arise.

HISTORY: Problem focused

EXAMINATION: Detailed

MEDICAL DECISION-MAKING: Low

TIME: 15 minutes spent with the patient; 5 minutes spent documenting in the EHR

Enter one diagnosis code and two procedure codes.

DX1

PR1

PR2

PRACTICE—SCENARIO 12

CHIEF COMPLAINT: Hematuria in a new patient

TIME OF EXAM ROOM ENTRY: 10:00 a.m.

HISTORY OF PRESENT ILLNESS: Patient is a 36-year-old female who presents to my office with acute onset of hematuria within the last 6 to 8 hours. However, over the past 2 days the patient has noted urinary pressure, urinary frequency, dysuria, and chills, although she denies any true rigors. She has not had any identifiable fever. She has mild low central abdominal discomfort but has had no nausea or vomiting. She has not noted changes in her bowel habits.

PAST MEDICAL HISTORY: Notable for arthritis in her right foot. There is no history of diabetes, ischemic heart disease, or hypertension. Has a significant history of schizophrenia.

SURGICAL HISTORY: She is status post corrective surgery on her right foot, status postoperative procedure on her cervix, and status post cyst removal at her right ankle.

CURRENT MEDICATIONS: Ibuprofen p.r.n.

ALLERGIES: Noted to PENICILLIN and SULFA

SOCIAL HISTORY: The patient lives independently. She smokes approximately 1/2 pack of cigarettes per day and denies excessive alcohol use.

REVIEW OF SYSTEMS:

GENERAL: Negative for any documented fevers, but the patient does report some chills. Her p.o. intake has been normal, and no weight loss described.

GI: See HPI

GU: See HPI

GYN: No unusual vaginal discharge or bleeding. The patient is sexually active. Does not believe she is pregnant.

PHYSICAL EXAMINATION:

VITAL SIGNS: Blood pressure 111/68; pulse is 86; respiration is 20; temperature is 97.8.

GENERAL: The patient is awake, alert, nontoxic, in no acute distress.

HEENT: Was unremarkable

NECK: Supple

LUNGS: Breath sounds clear and symmetric

CARDIAC: Regular S2, S2. No murmur or gallop appreciated.

ABDOMEN: Soft, nontender in the upper regions with some minimal suprapubic tenderness. There are no masses, organomegaly, or peritoneal signs present, and no tenderness present.

EXTREMITIES: No deformities, clubbing, or edema. Pulses full and symmetric throughout.

SKIN: Warm and dry. No jaundice, pallor, or cyanosis noted. No skin rash is present.

NEUROLOGIC: The patient is alert, fully oriented. Pupils equal, round, and reactive to light. The remainder of her examination is nonfocal.

PRACTICE—SCENARIO 12 (*continued*)

A voided urine specimen was obtained for pregnancy testing, and an automated urinalysis was done. Pregnancy test was negative, and the urinalysis demonstrated specific gravity of less than 1.005 with large occult blood and a large leukocyte esterase. Microscopy revealed 3 to 5 red blood cells were seen with greater than 100 red blood cells, and only an occasional squamous cell noted.

The results of her urinalysis and my findings and recommendations were discussed with the patient in detail. She was given Levaquin 500 mg orally in the office and a prescription for 5 additional days' worth. I recommended she drink plenty of fluids. Pyridium 100 mg, 1 to 2 q. 8 hours p.r.n. was prescribed for discomfort, and two tablets of Pyridium given to the patient for her use overnight. Patient was significantly agitated due to her ongoing schizophrenia. Patient was recommended to follow up with me in 3 to 5 days if not significantly improved.

TIME OF EXAM ROOM EXIT: 10:20 a.m.

DIAGNOSES: Acute urinary tract infection. Schizophrenia.

TOTAL TIME: I spent 20 minutes in the room with the patient, and 5 minutes documenting in the EHR after I exited the exam room.

Enter two diagnosis codes and three procedure codes.

___

DX1

DX2

PR1

PR2

PR3

PRACTICE—SCENARIO 13

DATE OF OPERATION: 09/25/20XX

PREOPERATIVE DIAGNOSES:

1. Left facial skin tag

2. Left preauricular sinus

POSTOPERATIVE DIAGNOSES:

1. Left facial skin tag

2. Left preauricular sinus

OPERATION:

1. Excision of left facial skin tag

2. Excision of left preauricular sinus tract with wound closure 1.1 cm

ANESTHESIA: General endotracheal anesthesia

FLUIDS: Approximately 100 cc crystalloid

ESTIMATED BLOOD LOSS: Less than 5 cc

URINE OUTPUT: None

CULTURES: None

DRAINS: None

SPECIMENS:

1. Left facial skin tag

2. Left preauricular sinus

FINDINGS: 1.1 cm left preauricular sinus and approximately 1 cm left facial skin tag

DESCRIPTION OF PROCEDURE: The patient was brought to the operating room. General endotracheal anesthesia was introduced. The table was turned 90° counterclockwise. The skin and subcutaneous tissue around the sinus, as well as the left facial skin tag, were infiltrated with 0.5% Marcaine with 1:100,000 epinephrine. A total of 1.5 cc was used. The patient was then prepared and draped in the usual sterile fashion.

Attention was first turned to the sinus and a lacrimal probe was used to determine the extent and direction of the sinus. The tract was approximately 1.1 cm, and the outline was made with a marking pen followed by incision through the skin and dermis with a Weck blade. Sharpie scissors were then used to dissect down to the sinus capsule and dissect out the capsule until it was removed and blocked. Hemostasis was then achieved, and the wound was closed in three layers; one to obliterate the subcutaneous tissues with 4-0 Vicryl simple interrupted followed by a single deep dermal of 4-0 Vicryl and finally the skin was reapproximated with a 6-0 fast absorbing gut running subcuticular suture.

Attention was then turned to the skin tag, and it was removed with a single snip of tenotomy scissors. The resulting wound was then reapproximated with a single 6-0 fast absorbing gut simple interrupted suture. The wound was dressed with Tegaderm and care of the patient returned to the anesthesia team.

COMPLICATIONS: None

DISPOSITION: To the postanesthesia care unit

PRACTICE—SCENARIO 13 (*continued*)

PATHOLOGY REPORT:

CLINICAL INFORMATION

PROCEDURE: Excision of left preauricular skin tag and sinus

PREOPERATIVE DIAGNOSIS: Preauricular skin tag and sinus, left

CLINICAL HISTORY: None given

GROSS DESCRIPTION:

1. Received in formalin for routine examination designated LEFT PREAURICULAR SINUS is a tan irregular fragment of tissue measuring 0.8 × 0.3 × 0.2 cm. The entire specimen is submitted in cassette A.

2. Received in formalin for routine examination designated SKIN TAG, LEFT PREAURICULAR is a cone-shaped fragment of tissue lined by skin measuring 0.5 cm in length with a variable diameter from 0.2 cm at the base to 0.1 cm at the tip. The cut margin is inked black. The specimen is bisected, wrapped, and submitted in cassette B.

MICROSCOPIC DESCRIPTION:

1. Microscopic sections examined; description omitted.

2. The facial skin tag is covered by keratinizing squamous epithelium with underlying intact adnexal structures and a central core of skeletal muscle.

DIAGNOSIS:

1. LEFT PREAURICULAR SINUS, EXCISION: DERMOID SINUS

2. LEFT PREAURICULAR SKIN TAG, EXCISION: HAMARTOMATOUS MALFORMATION OF SKIN AND SKELETAL MUSCLE. SEE COMMENT

COMMENT: Although the pathology requisition identifies the resected skin tag as coming from the left preauricular region, the clinic note from 8/24/20XX instead indicates that this skin tag was located posterolateral to the lateral canthus of the left eye.

Enter two diagnosis codes and three procedure codes.

DX1

DX2

PR1

PR2

PR3

PRACTICE—SCENARIO 14

DIAGNOSIS: s/p Tetralogy of Fallot repair

INDICATIONS: Palpitations

A two-channel Holter monitor was recorded for 23:59 hours. The predominant rhythm was sinus rhythm with sinus arrhythmia and wandering atrial pacemaker. Analysis of the recording revealed that the heart rate ranged from 70 to 145 bpm with an average heart rate of 99 bpm.

Supraventricular arrhythmias occurred. The mean frequency of supraventricular premature depolarizations was 0.7 beats per hour. The frequency ranged from 0 to 6 for a total of 16 beats. This represents <0.01% of the rhythm.

Supraventricular tachycardia occurred. 1 episode(s) occurred. The longest run was 3 beats. The fastest run was 118 bpm.

Ventricular arrhythmia did not occur. Ventricular couplets did not occur. Ventricular tachycardia did not occur. AV block did not occur. Bradycardia for patient's age was not recorded.

ECG INTERVALS: PR = 120–160 msec; QRS = 120 msec; QTc = 436–481 msec

No symptoms were recorded during the monitoring period.

IMPRESSION:

The quality of the tracing was good.

1. The predominant rhythm was normal sinus rhythm with sinus arrhythmia and wandering atrial pacemaker. Physiologic and circadian heart rate variation were mildly diminished. The heart rate ranged from 70 to 145 bpm, averaging 99 bpm.

2. Rare supraventricular premature beats occurred, comprising <0.01% of the total rhythm. There was 1 supraventricular couplet with a coupling interval of 0.560 msec.

3. Ventricular ectopy will not occur. Neither ventricular couplets nor runs occurred. VT did not occur.

4. Bradycardia did not occur. AV block did not occur.

5. No definite diagnosis identified.

Enter three diagnosis codes and one procedure code.

DX1

DX2

DX3

PR1

PRACTICE—SCENARIO 15

Please code for the services of the laboratory.

LABORATORY RESULTS

CLINICAL HISTORY: Hyperemesis gravidarum with electrolyte imbalance at 19 weeks' gestation

Drawn here today:

03/10/20XX 13:00 Basic Metabolic Panel for more Final Results Received				
Specimen Comment	1 SERUM SEPARATOR TUBE (SST)			Final
Sodium	137		[136–145 mmol/L]	Final
Potassium	3.3	L	[3.8–5.4 mmol/L]	Final
Chloride	95	L	[98–106 mmol/L]	Final
Carbon Dioxide	36	H	[20–26 mmol/L]	Final
BUN	14		[7–18 mg/dL]	Final
Creatinine	0.8		[0.4–1.0 mg/dL]	Final
Glucose	114	H	[70–106 mg/dL]	Final
Calcium (total)	7.7	L	[8.8–10.1 mg/dL]	Final

03/10/20XX 13:00 CBC with Auto Diff for more Final Results Received				
White Blood Cell Count	10.8		[4.5–13.5 THOU/μL]	Final
Red Blood Cell Count	3.56	L	[4.5–5.3 MIL/μL]	Final
Hemoglobin	10.8	L	[13.0–16.0 g/dL]	Final
Hematocrit	31.3	L	[37.0–49.0%]	Final
Mean Corpuscular Volume	87.8		[78.0–98.0 fL]	Final
Mean Corpuscular Hgb	30.4		[25.0–35.0 pg]	Final
Mean Corpus Hgb Conc	34.5		[31.0–37.0 g/dL]	Final
Red Distribution Width	15.7	H	[11.5–14.5%]	Final
Platelet Count	95	LL	[150–400 THOU/μL]	Final

CONSISTENT WITH PREVIOUS RESULTS				
Mean Platelet Volume	7.3	L	[7.4–10.4 fL]	Final
Segmented Neutrophils	95.7	H	[40–59%]	Final
Absolute Neutrophil Count	10,336		[THOU/μL]	Final
Eosinophils Count	0.6		[0–4%]	Final
Basophils	0		[0–1%]	Final
Lymphocytes	1.4	L	[34–48%]	Final
Monocytes	2.3	L	[3–8%]	Final
Platelet Estimate	Not Done			Final
Differential Method	AUTOMATED			Final

Enter one diagnosis code and three procedure codes.

DX1

PR1

PR2

PR3

PRACTICE—SCENARIO 16

DATE OF SERVICE: 12/29/20XX

CHIEF COMPLAINT: Acute left-sided weakness

HISTORY OF PRESENT ILLNESS: The patient is a 47-year-old female who was on the phone talking to a friend when she had acute weakness to her left arm and left leg. She states her leg and arm felt like an extremity feels when you sleep on it. There was decreased strength, but she states the symptoms and also the sensation is slightly decreased. Her husband noted some slight slurring of her speech. The patient denies any visual changes, loss of vision, double vision. She has not had any headache. She gives no history of any chest pain or palpitations. She presents here stating that her symptoms have somewhat improved.

PAST MEDICAL AND SURGICAL HISTORY:

1. Appendectomy
2. Mitral valve prolapse

CURRENT MEDICATIONS: Ranitidine

SOCIAL HISTORY: She does not smoke. She is a missionary. She has no primary care provider.

FAMILY HISTORY: Negative for early stroke or coronary artery disease.

REVIEW OF SYSTEMS: See HPI, otherwise negative.

PHYSICAL EXAMINATION:

VITAL SIGNS: Temperature 98.1; blood pressure 120/69; pulse 76 and regular, respirations 17; saturation 99% on room air

GENERAL: Awake, alert, non-toxic-appearing female

HEENT: Head is a traumatic, normocephalic. Pupils are equal and round. Extraocular muscles are intact. Cranial nerves II–XII are intact. The palate raises symmetrically.

NECK: Supple, no JVD, no bruits

CHEST: Clear and equal breath sounds bilaterally without any wheezes, rales, or rhonchi

CARDIOVASCULAR: S1 and S2 normal. Regular rate and rhythm. Occasional ectopic beat is noted. I do not appreciate any murmur.

ABDOMEN: Soft

EXTREMITIES: Warm and dry, well perfused

NEUROLOGICAL: She is awake, alert, oriented ×3. Her strength is 5/5 and symmetric. Finger-to-nose normal. Heel-to-shin normal.

EMERGENCY DEPARTMENT COURSE: The patient underwent extensive diagnostics. A continuous three-lead monitor demonstrated a sinus rhythm with occasional PVC. Twelve-lead electrocardiogram revealed a sinus rhythm, occasional PVC, no ST-segment elevation or depression. CT scan of her head was found to be unremarkable. Her white blood cell count was 4.7, normal hemoglobin and hematocrit, normal differential. Comprehensive metabolic and CK were all normal as well. The patient was given aspirin orally here in the department. Given that she is 47 years of age, has mitral valve prolapse, and has rather classic symptoms of a TIA and thought to be at high risk, the patient will be placed in the hospital for further inpatient workup for acute transient ischemic attack, which appears to be improved.

PRACTICE—SCENARIO 16 (*continued*)

DIAGNOSES:

1. Acute transient ischemic attack

2. Mitral valve prolapse by history

INSTRUCTIONS: The patient's case was discussed with cardiology. The patient will be admitted to a telemetry bed for further care and treatment.

HISTORY: Comprehensive

EXAMINATION: Comprehensive

MEDICAL DECISION-MAKING: High

Enter two diagnosis codes and two procedure codes.

DX1

DX2

PR1

PR2

PRACTICE—SCENARIO 17

HISTORY OF PRESENT ILLNESS: This is a 4-year-old Hispanic girl who is presenting new to me today and is 6 weeks after a left comminuted supracondylar fracture ×3, which occurred on 06/16/20XX status post closed reduction and percutaneous pinning by another physician on 06/17. The patient has Still's syndrome.

X-rays today show a well-healing fracture with pins in place. Long-arm cast was removed today prior to films.

Patient had pain for the first couple days after the injury and after the procedure and then patient denied pain. Her mom said that she had been complaining of pain after those first couple of days.

PAST MEDICAL HISTORY: She has no past medical history.

MEDICATIONS: No medications.

ALLERGIES: No allergies.

PHYSICAL EXAMINATION: On examination she has 3 percutaneous pins that are protruding from the dorsal aspect of the elbow. There are no signs of infection, no warmth, redness, or edema. She has normal sensation and motor function of the left hand and 2+ radial pulses.

IMPRESSION: Well-healing supracondylar fracture with percutaneous pins.

PLAN: Pins were removed today in clinic, and sterile dressing was applied. We will see this patient back in 4 weeks for follow-up with x-rays at that time. We counseled the mother regarding the limited activity for the patient over the next 4 weeks including no monkey bars, no running, no bicycling, and no activity where the patient would be at risk for a fall.

MEDICAL DECISION-MAKING: Low level

Enter two diagnosis codes and two procedure codes.

DX1

DX2

PR1

PR2

PRACTICE—SCENARIO 18

DATE OF OPERATION: 11/08/20XX

PREOPERATIVE DIAGNOSIS: Mucocele, inside right lower lip

POSTOPERATIVE DIAGNOSIS: Mucocele, inside right lower lip

OPERATION: Excision of right lower lip mucocele

ANESTHESIA: General via laryngeal mask airway (LMA)

SPECIMENS: Mucocele from right lower lip

OPERATIVE FINDINGS: Consistent with above

ESTIMATED BLOOD LOSS: Less than 10 mL

COMPLICATIONS: None

INDICATIONS: The patient is a healthy 6-year-old girl who was referred to our clinic from an outside medical clinic for evaluation of a lower lip mucocele. This small lesion has been present for several months and is indicated for removal. Prior to going to the operating room, the details of the procedure along with all risks and all questions were invited and answered with the mother with interpreter present. They elected to have this procedure performed in the operating room under general anesthesia.

PROCEDURE: The patient was properly identified in the preanesthesia holding area, and her consent, NPO status, and history and physical examination were updated, reviewed, and verified. At this time she was brought to operating theater #10 where she was placed in the supine position. Next, the anesthesia team induced and intubated the patient without complication. The tube was secured, and the patient was maintained under general anesthesia throughout the entire procedure. At this time a time-out and patient and procedure verification took place. Next, the patient was prepared, draped, and padded in the usual fashion for a procedure of this type. At this time approximately 2 cc of 0.25% Marcaine with epinephrine 1:200,000 was infiltrated in the right lower lip in the area of the medial nerve. Next, a #15 blade was used to make an elliptical incision around the 3 mm × 3 mm mucocele on the inside of the right lower lip. This was taken just through mucosa. Next, a superficial submucosal dissection was undertaken and the mucocele was removed in its entirety. The surgeon was careful to remain just under the mucosa so that no damage to the medial nerve or its branches would take place. Following this, the wound was irrigated and closed with 5-0 Vicryl in multiple running horizontal mattress sutures. The patient was then awakened, extubated, and taken to the postanesthesia care unit (PACU) in stable condition. There were no complications. All sponge and needle counts were correct ×2.

CLINICAL INFORMATION:

PROCEDURE: Excision of mucocele lower lip

PREOP DIAGNOSIS: Mucocele lower lip

CLINICAL HISTORY: Not given

GROSS DESCRIPTION: Received in formalin for routine examination designated MUCOCELE RIGHT LOWER LIP are two fragments of tissue measuring 0.6 cm and 0.2 cm in maximal dimension. The tissue is wrapped and entirely submitted in one cassette.

PRACTICE—SCENARIO 18 (*continued*)

PATHOLOGY REPORT:

MICROSCOPIC DESCRIPTION: Sections contain oral epithelium with underlying glandular tissue that has both serous and acinar cells. The gland has intact architecture, although lumen of the excretory duct is dilated. The stroma immediately under the oral epithelium contains an irregularly shaped cystic space that contains proteinaceous fluid and neutrophils. The adjacent stroma contains reactive capillaries and venules with mild chronic inflammation. No definite mucous is present. Additional step sections were examined.

DIAGNOSIS: ORAL MUCOSA, LOWER LIP, EXCISION: MUCOUS RETENTION CYST

Enter one diagnosis code and one procedure code.

DX1

PR1

PRACTICE—SCENARIO 19

DATE OF OPERATION: 12/08/20XX

PREOPERATIVE DIAGNOSES:

1. Stage IV metastatic renal cell carcinoma

2. Metastatic disease involving the left femoral neck, left peritrochanteric proximal femur with nondisplaced pathologic fracture of the neck of the femur

3. Metastatic disease involving the left supracondylar femur with impending pathologic fracture

PROCEDURE:

1. Resection of the left femoral head and metastatic neck, renal cell carcinoma

2. Long-stem cemented hemiarthroplasty utilizing the Smith & Nephew Echelon cemented 175-mm #12 stem with a 48-mm 0 neck endo-head

3. Extended curettage and methyl methaculate of the left supracondylar femur

4. Open reduction internal fixation of left distal femur utilizing a Synthes nine-hole 3.5 plate and screws

ANESTHESIA: General

ESTIMATED BLOOD LOSS: For the distal femur was less than 50 cc. For the hip was 150 cc.

INDICATIONS FOR PROCEDURE: This is a 58-year-old male in whom a large renal cell carcinoma was diagnosed earlier this year, who has undergone multiple other orthopedic procedures for bone disease, has had radiation therapy for a subtrochanteric lesion in the left femur, developed a new lytic lesion in the femoral neck, has gone on to progression and pain. Additionally, he was noted to have a separate discrete lesion in the distal supracondylar femur on the left. After preoperative embolization performed yesterday, the patient is brought to the operating room for the above-stated surgical procedures.

FINDINGS AT SURGERY: At the time of surgery, the left distal femur underwent an eventful curettage, methyl methaculate and open reduction internal fixation, given very stable fixation, ready for immediate weight bearing. The patient's proximal left femur was noted to have a nondisplaced but complete fracture at the base of the neck, therefore is not deemed a candidate for a spiral blade intermedullary fixation and therefore opted for a head and neck resection followed by a long-stemmed cemented hemiarthroplasty that also gave a very stable and excellent fixation ready for immediate weight bearing.

DESCRIPTION OF PROCEDURE: The patient was identified, brought to the operating room, and placed on the operating room table in the supine position, where general anesthesia was induced. The patient was oroendotracheally intubated. After he was stabilized, he was carefully and gently placed on the O.S.I. fracture table with a bump beneath the left hip. He received antibiotic prophylaxis, and the left hindquarter was prepared and draped in the usual sterile fashion. Under C-arm fluoroscopy, we ranged his hip and noted that the femoral head was not moving in unison with the femoral neck and therefore opted out of antegrade intermedullary nailing. We therefore proceeded with the distal femur first, which was approached with a direct lateral approach to the femur. The vastus lateralis was elevated. The underlying lytic lesion, which measured approximately 2 cm × 4 cm, was identified, entered with a sharp knife, then a burr, and curetted extensively throughout the intermedullary canal back to normal cortical bone. This was irrigated and dried with peroxide and saline. Methyl methaculate was mixed to a doughy state, digitally impacted to fill this defect. A nine-hole 3.5 Synthes plate was then bent and twisted to contour the lateral femur and fixed in the usual standard fashion with 35 screws. This gave excellent rigid fixation. Routine closure was obtained utilizing 0, 2-0 Vicryl followed by skin staples and sterile Tegaderm.

PRACTICE—SCENARIO 19 (*continued*)

At this time the patient was again prepared and draped in the right lateral decubitus position with care taken to pad bony prominences, neurovascular structures for a posterior approach to his left hip. Through a standard posterolateral approach to his hip, the proximal femur was identified, hip arthrotomy performed, and findings as noted above osteotomizing the proximal femur just above the lesser trochanter. Femoral head and neck were excised and found to be extensively involved with malignancy. These were passed off as specimen. The proximal femur was curetted back to stable bone. Then it was reamed and broached to accept a 175-mm #12 stem. Length was verified as satisfactory under C-arm fluoroscopy. The canal was prepared, dried, distal cement restrictor placed, and the #12 stem was cemented into standard anteversion utilizing excellent cement technique. After it had dried, a 48-mm 0 neck was impacted onto the prosthesis having been previously measured. This was reduced and noted to give excellent stable reduction. The wound was then copiously irrigated with antibiotic-containing saline solution and closed with 0 Vicryl interrupted, short external rotators reattached to the gluteus medius tendon, fascia closed with 0 Vicryl interrupted, 2-0 Vicryl inverted and skin staples. A medium Hemovac drain was used in the hip wound.

The patient was then returned to the supine position, awakened and extubated in the operating room, and moved to the recovery room in stable condition.

POSTOPERATIVE PLAN: For routine posterior hip precautions, weight bearing as tolerated.

Enter three diagnosis codes and three procedure codes.

DX1

DX2

DX3

PR1

PR2

PR3

PRACTICE—SCENARIO 20

DATE OF OPERATION: 12/15/20XX

PREOPERATIVE DIAGNOSIS: Right middle ear cholesteatoma

POSTOPERATIVE DIAGNOSIS: Right middle ear cholesteatoma

OPERATION: Right mastoidectomy, tympanoplasty

FINDINGS: Cholesteatoma, right anterior middle ear epitympanum, intact ossicular chain

INDICATIONS: The patient is an 18-year-old female with previous ear surgery elsewhere and then a right tympanoplasty here in 2001 for anterior-superior middle ear cholesteatoma. She was seen recently with enlarging right anterior-superior whitish mass within the tympanic membrane.

OPERATIVE PROCEDURE: After endotracheal intubation and administration of general anesthesia, the right ear was prepared and draped in the usual fashion. The ear was inspected with a microscope. The patient was known to have a whitish mass within an intact tympanic membrane in the anterior-superior quadrant of the middle ear. A canal incision was made 4 mm behind the posterior bony annulus with a 7200 blade from 6 o'clock to 12 o'clock. A postauricular incision was made with a #15 blade knife, and the periosteum was divided under the linea temporalis and behind the ear canal. At this point, the patient was found to have no accessible temporalis fascia. The temporalis muscle was then retracted superiorly with a Senn rake, and a 1.5 cm × 1.5 cm periosteal graft was harvested from underneath the temporalis fascia. This was cleaned and placed on the Mayo stand for drying. The ear canal was brought forward with a Freer elevator down to the previously made incision.

At this point, the patient was known to have a cholesteatoma that was within the posterior-superior ear canal in an area of scalloped-out bone. This cholesteatoma pearl was removed with a duckbill and then stapes curette. This was not contiguous with any other process. The tympanomeatal flap was elevated down to bony annulus, and then the middle ear was entered under the membranous annulus with a Rosen needle and annulus elevator. It was reflected forward to the malleus handle. At this point, the patient was known to have cholesteatoma extending along the medial surface of the malleus handle and body of malleus involving the anterior portion of tensor tympani tendon and filling the entire anterior middle ear and anterior epitympanum. The tympanic membrane was dissected off the malleus handle in its entirety with a 5910 Beaver blade and then reflected up to the anterior ear canal. The cholesteatoma mass was removed from the anterior hypotympanum, anterior-superior middle ear, and anterior epitympanum with a combination of duckbills and cupped forceps. It was difficult to visualize the tensor tympani tendon. The tensor tympani tendon was therefore cut at its attachment to the neck of the malleus with a 5910 blade and, with gentle lateral retraction on the malleus, the cholesteatoma could be followed up and dissected off the anterior surface of the body of the malleus. At this point, no other cholesteatoma was noted in the middle ear or epitympanum.

A mastoidectomy was carried out by removing the lateral cortex with a 3-mm burr to expose the posterior epitympanum. Dissection was carried further up to the short process of the malleus with a stapes curette. The mucosa in the posterior epitympanum was clean. No other cholesteatoma was noted under the incus. Irrigation at that point flowed freely over the facial ridge into the middle ear.

PRACTICE—SCENARIO 20 (*continued*)

Next, the middle ear was inspected again. A small amount of granulation tissue was dissected from around the long process of the incus and the incudostapedial joint, which was intact. No cholesteatoma was noted in that area. At this point, inspection of the middle ear and epitympanum yielded no evidence of recurrent cholesteatoma. A portion of the anterior tympanic membrane from the malleus handle up to the annulus was resected, where that had been contiguous with the main portion of the inflamed cholesteatoma mass. This resulted in about a 35% anterior marginal perforation. The anterior annulus was raised at the level of the perforation with a round 90-degree canal knife, and a Rosen needle was then used to make an adjacent tunnel under anterior ear canal skin. The previously harvested periosteal graft was placed under the malleus handle so that the anterior edge was positioned just at the mouth of the eustachian tube. A microcup forceps was placed into the previously made tunnel, and the anterior edge of the graft was pulled up anterior and underneath the anterior membranous annulus in order to hold the graft in place on the anterior canal wall. The posterior aspect of the graft and the tympanomeatal flap were reflected forward, and several pieces of Gelfoam were placed in the middle ear and pushed forward, and the graft was elevated to meet the surrounding tympanic membrane. The posterior aspect of the graft was placed on the posterior ear canal along the remainder of the tympanomeatal flap, and Gelfoam was placed starting anteriorly to reconstitute the anterior sulcus and then over the entire tympanic membrane and graft.

The postauricular incision was closed in three layers with periosteum, auricular muscle, and dermis with 3-0 and 4-0 chromic. Steri-Strips were applied, and Gelfoam was then used to pack the remainder of the external ear canal. Estimated blood loss was approximately 100 cc. The final status of the middle ear is intact mobile ossicular chain, medial periosteal graft to anterior marginal 35% perforation.

PLAN: I explained to the patient's parents that if we get a significant recurrence along the ossicles, then the plan in the future will probably be to divide the incudostapedial joint and remove the head of the malleus and incus for better access to the epitympanum.

Enter one diagnosis code and one procedure code.

DX1

PR1

CCS-P

EXAM 1

For the following questions, choose the best answer. A blank answer sheet for these multiple-choice questions can be found on page 56.

Domain 1 *Diagnosis Coding*

1. The physician visits his patient in the hospital and indicates that the patient has diabetes. Insulin is prescribed for and administered to the patient. What is the best decision that the coding professional can make in this situation?

   a. Assign a code for type 1 diabetes mellitus because insulin was administered.

   b. Assign a code for drug-induced diabetes mellitus.

   c. Assign a code for type 2 diabetes mellitus with complications.

   d. Assign a code for type 2 diabetes mellitus along with a code for the insulin use.

2. The patient is seen in the emergency department (ED) with acute lumbar pain. The ED physician documents possible kidney stones and orders an x-ray. The radiologist documents bilateral nephrolithiasis. The coding professional would assign a code for which of the following conditions?

   a. Acute lumbar pain

   b. Bilateral nephrolithiasis

   c. Possible kidney stones

   d. Abnormal x-ray findings

3. A female infant was born in the hospital at term and at a normal birth weight. It was a vaginal delivery with a vertex presentation. In the hours after birth, jaundice was noted and eventually a diagnosis of erythroblastosis fetalis due to an ABO incompatibility was made. How would this admission be coded?

Z38.00	Single liveborn, born in hospital, delivered vaginally
P55.0	Rh isoimmunization of newborn
P55.1	ABO isoimmunization of newborn
P55.8	Other hemolytic diseases of newborn
P55.9	Hemolytic disease of newborn, unspecified

   a. Z38.00, P55.0

   b. Z38.00, P55.1

   c. Z38.00, P55.8

   d. Z38.00, P55.9

4. The patient is seen in his ophthalmologist's office and treated for bilateral open angle glaucoma, moderate stage. How would this encounter be coded?

> | H40.10X2 | Unspecified open-angle glaucoma, moderate stage |
> |----------|--|
> | H40.1111 | Primary open-angle glaucoma, right eye, mild stage |
> | H40.1112 | Primary open-angle glaucoma, right eye, moderate stage |
> | H40.9 | Unspecified glaucoma |

   a. H40.10X2

   b. H40.1111

   c. H40.9

   d. H40.1112

5. **Inpatient admission:** The patient is a 78-year-old female with heart palpitations and abdominal pain who was brought to the ED by her grandson. The physician ordered an EKG, a complete blood count, and upper GI series. The GI revealed significant gastritis. The EKG was not significantly abnormal. The CBC revealed the following: Hct 23%; Hgb 6.5; and WBC 6,000. The cardiologist who admitted the patient into the hospital indicated he felt the palpitations were a symptom of the patient's significant anemia. Social services were notified because the physician felt that the patient was not receiving the proper nutritional support causing the hemoglobin deficiency. The patient received 2 units of packed cells and was discharged the following day. The discharge diagnoses included nutritional anemia and gastritis. What codes would be reported for this encounter?

   a. D53.9, K29.70

   b. D53.9, K29.70, R00.2

   c. D53.9, K29.70, R10.9

   d. D53.9, K29.70, R00.2, R10.9

6. A 77-year-old white female is seen with interstitial pneumonitis. Hospital course here has been complicated by hypoxemia, renal insufficiency, and steroid-induced diabetes mellitus. The patient has been taking steroids as prescribed for quite some time for her rheumatoid arthritis. The patient reports having episodes of small volume painless hematochezia at home secondary to hemorrhoids. Last evening and this morning, the patient experienced larger volume bright red blood per rectum. The patient reports having a colonoscopy about three years ago performed elsewhere revealing diverticulosis and hemorrhoids. She states she had sequential colonoscopies performed in the past. However, she is unclear on the findings.

Final Diagnoses Upon Discharge:

1. Hematochezia

2. Interstitial pneumonitis

3. Steroid-induced diabetes mellitus

4. Chronic renal insufficiency

5. Hypoxemia

What codes are reported for this condition?

   a. E11.9, J84.9, R09.02, K92.1, M06.9, N18.9, T38.0X5A, Z79.4

   b. E09.9, J84.9, R09.02, K92.1, M06.9, N18.9, T38.0X5A

   c. E09.9, J84.9, K92.1, M06.9, N18.6, T38.0X5A

   d. E09.9, J84.9, K92.1, M06.9, N18.9, T38.0X5A

7. Using the following illustration from the Table of Drugs and Chemicals in the ICD-10-CM code book, which code would a coding professional select for the following diagnosis: "Initial presentation for excessive drowsiness due to sensitivity to Periactin taken as prescribed"?

Table of Drugs and Chemicals						
Substance	Poisoning, Accidental	Poisoning, Intentional	Poisoning, Assault	Poisoning, Undetermined	Adverse Effect	Underdosing
Periactin	T45.0x1	T45.0x2	T45.0x3	T45.0x4	T45.0x5	T45.0x6
Note: 7th character "A" is assigned to indicate initial encounter.						

a. T45.0X2A

b. T45.0X6A

c. T45.0X4A

d. T45.0X5A

8. A patient visits his physician's office and indicates that he has left arm paralysis due to a case of poliomyelitis that he suffered as a young child. What diagnosis codes would be assigned for this diagnosis?

A80.9	Acute poliomyelitis, unspecified
B91	Sequelae of poliomyelitis
G81.90	Hemiplegia, unspecified affecting unspecified side
G83.20	Monoplegia of upper limb affecting unspecified side
G83.22	Monoplegia of upper limb affecting left dominant side
G83.24	Monoplegia of upper limb affecting left nondominant side

a. G83.24, B91

b. B91, G83.22

c. G81.90, A80.9

d. B91, G83.20

9. A 26-year-old female delivers a 36-week, full-term infant per the physician's documentation. The young mother has been previously diagnosed with AIDS. What is the correct diagnosis code assignment for the physician's services?

O98.72	Human immunodeficiency virus [HIV] disease complicating childbirth
B20	Human immunodeficiency virus [HIV] disease
O60.14X0	Preterm labor third trimester with preterm delivery third trimester, not applicable or unspecified
Z37.0	Single live birth
Z21	Asymptomatic human immunodeficiency virus [HIV] infection status
Z3A.36	36 weeks gestation of pregnancy

a. O98.72, O60.14X0, B20, Z37.0, Z3A.36

b. O98.72, B20, Z37.0, Z3A.36

c. O98.72, Z21, Z37.0, Z3A.36

d. O98.72, O60.14X0, Z21, Z3A.36

10. In which of the following situations would acute respiratory failure be considered as the secondary diagnosis?

    a. A patient with emphysema develops acute respiratory failure and is admitted for treatment.

    b. A patient with congestive heart failure is brought to the ED in acute respiratory failure and is intubated and admitted.

    c. A patient overdoses on crack cocaine and is admitted to the hospital in acute respiratory failure.

    d. A patient with chronic myasthenia gravis suffers an acute exacerbation and develops acute respiratory failure. The patient is admitted to treat the respiratory failure.

11. A patient is admitted with MRSA pneumonia. The physician also documents MRSA colonization. What codes are reported for this admission?

A49.02	Methicillin resistant Staphylococcus aureus infection, unspecified site
J15.212	Pneumonia due to Methicillin resistant Staphylococcus aureus
Z22.322	Carrier or suspected carrier of Methicillin resistant Staphylococcus aureus

    a. A49.02, Z22.322

    b. J15.212, A49.02, Z22.322

    c. J15.212

    d. J15.212, Z22.322

12. The patient is admitted to the hospital for a third round of chemotherapy for her acute lymphoblastic leukemia. On the second day of hospitalization, the patient develops severe nausea and vomiting. Which of the following codes would be reported as the principal diagnosis?

    a. Z51.11, Encounter for antineoplastic chemotherapy

    b. C91.00, Acute lymphoblastic leukemia not having achieved remission

    c. R11.2, Nausea with vomiting, unspecified

    d. Z51.12, Encounter for antineoplastic immunotherapy

13. The patient was seen today for a postsurgical wound infection (*Escherichia coli*) with intra-muscular abscess following surgery for an open, type 1, right tibial shaft fracture. There is routine healing of the fracture. Which of the following diagnosis codes would be reported by the physician?

    a. T81.41XA, B96.21, S82.201E

    b. T81.42XA, B96.20, S82.201S

    c. T81.42XA, B96.20, S82.201E

    d. T81.41XD, B96.20, S82.201E

14. The physician sees a patient in the hospital with a diagnosis of "metastasis to the brain admitted in a comatose state." In ICD-10-CM, how would this diagnosis be coded?

    a. Code only the brain metastasis (C79.31) with unknown primary site (C80.1).

    b. Code only the unknown primary site (C80.1).

    c. Code the metastasis (C79.31) followed by a code for the coma (R40.20) and unknown primary site (C80.1).

    d. Code only the coma (R40.20).

15. The patient is seen in the wound clinic with bilateral decubitus ulcers of the buttocks. The physician documents the stage of the ulcers as stage 3. What diagnosis codes would be submitted for this encounter?

L89.313	Pressure ulcer of right buttock, stage 3
L89.323	Pressure ulcer of left buttock, stage 3
L89.303	Pressure ulcer of unspecified buttock, stage 3
L89.43	Pressure ulcer of contiguous site of back, buttock and hip, stage 3

    a. L89.313, L89.323

    b. L89.313, L89.313

    c. L89.43, L89.303

    d. L89.323, L89.323

16. A liveborn infant was born vaginally in the hospital and shortly thereafter was diagnosed with fetal alcohol syndrome. The infant's mother was alcohol dependent. How would this case be coded?

    a. Z38.00, Q86.0

    b. Z38.01, Q86.0

    c. Z38.00, F10.20

    d. Z38.01, F10.20

Domain 2   *Procedure Coding*

17. Wide excision of a 0.65-cm malignant melanoma (margins included) from right forearm. Which of the following diagnosis and procedure codes are reported?

C43.61	Malignant melanoma of right upper limb, including shoulder
C76.41	Malignant neoplasm of right upper limb
11401	Excision, benign lesion including margins, except skin tag (unless listed elsewhere), trunk, arms, or legs; excised diameter 0.6 to 1.0 cm
11601	Excision, malignant lesion including margins, trunk, arms, or legs; excised diameter 0.6 to 1.0 cm
25075	Excision, tumor, soft tissue of forearm and/or wrist area, subcutaneous; less than 3 cm

a. C76.41, 11401

b. C76.41, 11601

c. C43.61, 11601

d. C43.61, 25075

18. The physician performs therapeutic injections of both the patient's facet joints at L1–L2 and L2-L3, using fluoroscopic guidance. How is this coded?

64490	Injection(s), diagnostic or therapeutic agent, paravertebral facet (zygapophyseal) joint (or nerves innervating that joint) with image guidance (fluoroscopy or CT), cervical or thoracic; single level
64493	Injection(s), diagnostic or therapeutic agent, paravertebral facet (zygapophyseal) joint (or nerves innervating that joint) with image guidance (fluoroscopy or CT), lumbar or sacral; single level
64494	second level (List separately in addition to code for primary procedure)
64495	third and any additional level(s) (List separately in addition to code for primary procedure)
-50	Bilateral procedure

a. 64493-50, 64494-50

b. 64490-50, 64494-50

c. 64493, 64493

d. 64495

19. The physician performs a median sternotomy and places the patient on cardiopulmonary bypass to repair the patient's aortopulmonary window, or a connection between the aorta and pulmonary artery just above the semilunar valves. The physician opens the pulmonary artery and locates the window, closing it with a Dacron fabric patch. The patient is taken off bypass, and the sternal incision is closed. How is this procedure coded?

a. 33645, Direct or patch closure, sinus venosus, with or without anomalous pulmonary venous drainage

b. 33813, Obliteration of aortopulmonary septal defect; without cardiopulmonary bypass

c. 33814, Obliteration of aortopulmonary septal defect; with cardiopulmonary bypass

d. 33917, Repair of pulmonary artery stenosis by reconstruction with patch or graft

20. The physician orders the following blood tests, which are performed together at the office: Carbon dioxide, Chloride, Potassium, Sodium. How are these tests coded?

80051	Electrolyte panel: Carbon dioxide (bicarbonate); Chloride; Potassium; Sodium
80053	Comprehensive metabolic panel: Albumin; Bilirubin, total; Calcium, total; Carbon dioxide (bicarbonate); Chloride; Creatinine; Glucose; Phosphatase, alkaline; Potassium; Protein, total; Sodium; Transferase, alanine amino (ALT) (SGPT); Transferase, aspartate amino (AST)(SGOT); Urea nitrogen (BUN)
82374	Carbon dioxide (bicarbonate)
82435	Chloride; blood
82436	Chloride; urine
84132	Potassium; serum, plasma or whole blood
84133	Potassium; urine
84295	Sodium; serum, plasma or whole blood
84302	Sodium; other source

a. 82374, 82435, 84132, 84295

b. 82374, 82436, 84133, 84302

c. 80051

d. 80053

21. The patient has L2–3 spinal stenosis. The surgeon removes the lower portion of the L2 spinous process and the upper portion of the L3 spinous process, as well as the interspinous ligament to provide access to the space. A spinous process distraction device is then inserted using imaging guidance. How is this service coded?

22102	Partial excision of posterior vertebral component (eg, spinous process, lamina or facet) for intrinsic bony lesion, single vertebral segment, lumbar
22612	Arthrodesis, posterior or posterolateral technique, single interspace; lumbar (with lateral transverse technique, when performed)
22841	Internal spinal fixation by wiring of spinous processes (List separately in addition to code for primary procedure)
22869	Insertion of interlaminar/interspinous process stabilization/distraction device, without open decompression or fusion, including image guidance when performed, lumbar; single level

a. 22102, 22841

b. 22612, 22841

c. 22869

d. 22102, 22869

22. An infant is born with a large gastroschisis. The intestines are mechanically eased into the abdomen using a prosthesis. Surgical closure is completed after one week. What is the correct CPT coding for the final closure?

    a. 49600, Repair of small omphalocele, with primary closure

    b. 49605, Repair of large omphalocele or gastroschisis; with or without prosthesis

    c. 49606, Repair of large omphalocele or gastroschisis; with removal of prosthesis, final reduction and closure, in operating room

    d. 49611, Repair of omphalocele (Gross type operation); second stage

23. The patient undergoes a completely thoracoscopic, off-pump coronary artery bypass procedure using a daVinci robot. Three ports are placed in the thorax for the robotic arms and the camera. The physician uses the system to obtain the internal mammary artery and graft it to the left anterior descending coronary artery. How is this procedure coded?

    a. 33533

    b. 33533, 33999

    c. 33534

    d. 33999

24. The patient undergoes a vaginal hysterectomy with a 230-gram uterus, bilateral salpingectomy, and unilateral oophorectomy. How is this coded?

    a. 58260, 58720

    b. 58260, 58700-50, 58940

    c. 58262

    d. 58285

25. The patient had a total ethmoidectomy five days ago and now presents with headache and a clear nasal discharge. The surgeon performs a nasal endoscopy looking for a CSF leak and repairs the leak at the prior procedure site. What is the correct code assignment for this repair?

    a. 31238

    b. 31290

    c. 31291

    d. 31299

26. The physician curettes three lesions off the patient's back. The lesions are keratotic and measure 0.5 cm each. How is this service coded?

11400	Excision, benign lesion including margins, except skin tag (unless listed elsewhere), trunk, arms, or legs; excised diameter 0.5 cm or less
11402	excised diameter 1.1 to 2.0 cm
17000	Destruction (eg, laser surgery, electrosurgery, cryosurgery, chemosurgery, surgical curettement), premalignant lesions (eg, actinic keratoses); first lesion
+17003	second through 14 lesions, each (List separately in addition to code for first lesion)
-51	Multiple procedures

a. 11400, 11400-51, 11400-51

b. 11402

c. 17000

d. 17000, 17003 × 2

27. A 9-year-old boy is seen in the emergency department and receives 560 units of rabies immune globulin and rabies vaccine as intramuscular injections after being bitten by a squirrel that exhibited signs of being infected. The documentation contains an expanded problem-focused history, a detailed examination, and high-level medical decision-making. How are these services coded?

99283	Emergency department visit for the evaluation and management of a patient, which requires these 3 key components: an expanded problem focused history; an expanded problem focused examination; and medical decision making of moderate complexity
99284	Emergency department visit for the evaluation and management of a patient, which requires these 3 key components: a detailed history; a detailed examination; and medical decision making of moderate complexity
99285	Emergency department visit for the evaluation and management of a patient, which requires these 3 key components within the constraints imposed by the urgency of the patient's clinical condition and/or mental status: a comprehensive history; a comprehensive examination; and medical decision making of high complexity
90375	Rabies immune globulin (RIg), human, for intramuscular and/or subcutaneous use
90471	Immunization administration (includes percutaneous, intradermal, subcutaneous, or intramuscular injections); 1 vaccine (single or combination vaccine/toxoid)
90675	Rabies vaccine, for intramuscular use
90676	Rabies vaccine, for intradermal use
96372	Therapeutic, prophylactic, or diagnostic injection (specify substance or drug); subcutaneous or intramuscular

a. 99283, 90676, 90675

b. 99283, 90375, 90675, 90471, 96372

c. 99284, 90375 × 560 units, 90675, 96372 × 2

d. 99285, 90375, 90676, 90471, 96372

28. A patient presents to Dr. Smith's office reporting fever, chills, and a productive cough. Dr. Smith admits her to the hospital later that same day. What E/M service(s) would Dr. Smith bill for?

    a. Outpatient visit and an initial hospital care

    b. No E/M code can be submitted for that day

    c. Initial hospital care

    d. Only the outpatient visit

29. Preventive medicine services are based upon which of the following criteria?

    a. The final diagnosis for the visit

    b. Age of the patient

    c. Documentation of history, physical examination, and medical decision-making

    d. Amount of time spent with the patient

30. Physician A saw a patient in the morning and provided 50 minutes of critical care service. Physician B, who is Physician A's colleague from the same group, saw the patient later the same day and provided 35 minutes of critical care services. How would this be reported by the facility?

    a. Code 99291 would be used for the initial time (up to 74 minutes) and one unit of 99292 for the remaining time.

    b. Code 99291 would be the only code reported.

    c. Code 99292 would be the only code reported.

    d. Code 99291 would be used twice—once to reflect Dr. A's time and once to reflect Dr. B's time.

31. An established patient presents to the gastroenterologist with complaints of abdominal pain. The physician documents a detailed history, a detailed examination, that he spent 5 minutes reviewing records from the primary physician, that he spent 15 minutes in the room with the patient, and that he spent 5 minutes documenting in the EHR. Which E/M code should be used for reporting this service?

    a. 99202

    b. 99203

    c. 99212

    d. 99213

32. A patient is seen in the emergency department (ED) with acute appendicitis. The surgeon sees the patient, makes a diagnosis, and reaches a decision to perform surgery. The patient then has a laparoscopic appendectomy. How would the surgeon report this encounter?

    a. Code 44970 for laparoscopic appendectomy

    b. Code 44970 and a code from ED services

    c. Code 44970 and a code from ED services with a modifier to indicate reason for surgery

    d. Code 44970 with a modifier for increased procedural service

33. A 78-year-old male has a stage 3 pressure ulcer on the sacrum. The ulcer is excised and closed with myocutaneous flaps, transferred from the left and right buttocks. How is this service coded?

    a. 15934, 15734

    b. 15934, 15738

    c. 15936, 15734, 15734-59

    d. 15936, 15756, 15756-59

34. **In-Office Chemotherapy Administration**

    The patient is a 73-year-old female who arrives today for her scheduled chemotherapy treatment. All injections are sequential.

    Treatment today:

    Carboplatin infusion, 50 mg
       Start time 1:30 p.m., End time 2:05 p.m.
    Paclitaxel infusion, 25 mg
       Start time 2:06 p.m., End time 3:10 p.m.
    Ondansetron infusion, 1 mg
       Start time 3:12 p.m., End time 3:32 p.m.

    a. 96365, 96366, 96372, J2405, J9045, J9267 × 25

    b. 96413, 96417, 96368, J2405, J9045, J9267

    c. 96413, 96417, 96367

    d. 96413, 96417, 96367, J2405, J9045, J9267 × 25

35. The physician treats a patient who has osteomyelitis of the left shoulder blade following a past injury. A piece of dead bone is removed from the body of the shoulder blade, and the physician removes surrounding bone to return the shoulder blade to its natural contour. How is this coded?

23140	Excision or curettage of bone cyst or benign tumor of clavicle or scapula
23170	Sequestrectomy (eg, for osteomyelitis or bone abscess), clavicle
23172	Sequestrectomy (eg, for osteomyelitis or bone abscess), scapula
23180	Partial excision (craterization, saucerization, or diaphysectomy) bone (eg, osteomyelitis), clavicle
23182	Partial excision (craterization, saucerization, or diaphysectomy) bone (eg, osteomyelitis), scapula
23190	Ostectomy of scapula, partial (eg, superior medial angle)
-LT	Left side

    a. 23170-LT, 23140-51-LT

    b. 23172-LT, 23140-51-LT

    c. 23172-LT, 23182-51-LT

    d. 23190-LT, 23180-51-LT

36. When coding repairs of multiple lacerations in CPT, what action should the coding professional take?

    a. Code only the most complex repair.

    b. Code only the least complex repair.

    c. Code all the laceration repairs, listing the most complex repair first.

    d. Code all the repairs of the same site using the code for the most complex repair.

37. A patient underwent PTCA with stent in the left anterior descending artery, followed by atherectomy with stent in the left circumflex. How would this be coded?

    a. 92928-LD, 92933-LC

    b. 92928-LD, 92934-LC

    c. 92933-LC, 92928-LD

    d. 92933-LC, 92929-LD

38. After completion of allergy testing, the allergist prepares and provides allergenic extracts in 20 single-dose vials to begin desensitization. These vials are sent to the patient's primary care physician, who will administer the injections according to the prescribed schedule. How are the services of the allergist coded?

95117	Professional services for allergen immunotherapy not including provision of allergenic extracts; 2 or more injections
95144	Professional services for the supervision of preparation and provision of antigens for allergen immunotherapy, single dose vial(s) (specify number of vials)
95165	Professional services for the supervision of preparation and provision of antigens for allergen immunotherapy; single or multiple antigens (specify number of doses)
95199	Unlisted allergy/clinical immunologic service or procedure

   a. 95117×10

   b. 95144×20

   c. 95165×20

   d. 95199

39. A 60-year-old female calls the physician's office saying she was billed for a "male" shot, saying "I always get the same thing." The claim for that date shows 1 unit of J1071 was billed, with diagnoses of Z79.890 and N95.2. The encounter form for the visit states "Estrogen therapy." What error does the coding manager suspect?

J1050	Injection, medroxyprogesterone acetate, 1 mg
J1071	Injection, testosterone cypionate, 1 mg
Z79.890	Hormone replacement therapy
N95.2	Postmenopausal atrophic vaginitis

   a. The coding professional chose a code for the wrong medication.

   b. The coding professional chose a code for the wrong dosage of medication.

   c. The coding professional assumed that estradiol was administered at that visit.

   d. The coding professional reported an incorrect diagnosis code for the service.

40. To correctly code a total thyroidectomy, what vital piece of information must be documented to support code assignment?

   a. Whether parathyroid glands are excised

   b. Whether a surgical drain was placed

   c. Reason for thyroidectomy

   d. Surgical approach

41. According to the National Correct Coding Initiative guidelines, if a physician submits two codes of an edit pair:

    a. Neither code is payable.

    b. The column two code is not payable.

    c. The column two code may be payable with a PTP-associated modifier.

    d. The column two code will be considered medically unlikely.

42. A patient presents for removal of a pilonidal cyst. The physician must first perform an incision and drainage of the pilonidal cyst, before performing an extensive excision of the lesion. How would this be coded?

    a. 10081

    b. 11770, 10081

    c. 11771

    d. 11771, 10081

43. A patient is seen in the emergency department following an accident. The physician documents that the wound repair required multiple layers and extensive undermining. According to CPT definitions, this type of repair would be classified as:

    a. Simple

    b. Intermediate

    c. Complex

    d. Advancement

44. A patient undergoes excision of a 2 cm × 2 cm benign lesion on the left arm that the physician repairs with rotational flap. How would this be coded?

11402	Excision, benign lesion including margins, except skin tag (unless listed elsewhere), trunk, arms or legs, excised diameter 1.1 to 2.0 cm
14000	Adjacent tissue transferor rearrangement, trunk; defect 10 sq cm or less
14020	Adjacent tissue transfer or rearrangement, scalp, arms and/or legs; defect 10 sq cm or less

    a. 11402

    b. 11402, 14020

    c. 14020

    d. 14000

45. A patient presents to the ambulatory surgery center for a diagnostic esophagogastroduodenoscopy. During the procedure, the physician performs a balloon dilation. How would this be coded?

43235	Esophagogastroduodenoscopy, flexible, transoral; diagnostic, including collection of specimen(s) by brushing or washing, when performed (separate procedure)
43249	with transendoscopic balloon dilation of esophagus (less than 30 mm diameter)
43450	Dilation of esophagus, by unguided sound or bougie, single or multiple passes

    a. 43235, 43249

    b. 43235, 43450

    c. 43249

    d. 43450

46. A patient undergoes a split thickness autograft from the back to the arm. The donor site is repaired with simple sutures. The arm lesion measures 9 cm by 20 cm. How would this procedure be coded?

12005	Simple repair of superficial wounds of scalp, neck, axillae, external genitalia, trunk and/or extremities (including hands and feet); 12.6 cm to 20.0 cm
15040	Harvest of skin for tissue cultured skin autograft; 100 sq cm or less
15100	Split-thickness autograft, trunk, arms, legs; first 100 sq cm or less, or 1% of body surface area of infants and children (except 15050)
+15101	each additional 100 sq cm, or each additional 1% of body area of infants and children, or part thereof (List separately in addition to code for primary procedure)

    a. 15100, 15040, 12005

    b. 15100, 15101, 15040, 12005

    c. 15100

    d. 15100, 15101

47. A 12-year-old boy presents to the ER with groin pain. He is diagnosed with an inguinal hernia. The physician repairs the reducible hernia, including implantation of mesh. How would this procedure be coded?

49505	Repair initial inguinal hernia, age 5 years or older; reducible
49520	Repair recurrent inguinal hernia, any age; reducible
+49568	Implantation of mesh or other prosthesis for open incisional or ventral hernia repair or mesh for closure of debridement for necrotizing soft tissue infection (List separately in addition to code for the incisional or ventral hernia repair)

    a. 49505

    b. 49505, 49568

    c. 49520

    d. 49520, 49568

48. The physician performs a therapeutic thoracoscopic wedge resection of the lung. How would this procedure be coded?

32480	Removal of lung, other than pneumonectomy; single lobe (lobectomy)
32505	Thoracotomy, with therapeutic wedge resection (eg, mass, nodule), initial
32607	Thoracoscopy; with diagnostic biopsy(ies) of lung infiltrate(s) (eg, wedge, incisional), unilateral
32666	Thoracoscopy, surgical; with therapeutic wedge resection (eg, mass, nodule), initial unilateral

    a. 32480

    b. 32505

    c. 32607

    d. 32666

Domain 3 *Research*

49. A patient undergoes surgical insertion of a uterus harvested from a cadaver donor. How is this coded?

57155	Insertion of a uterine tandem and/or vaginal ovoids for clinical brachytherapy
58999	Unlisted procedure, female genital system (nonobstetrical)
0664T	Donor hysterectomy; open, from cadaver donor
0667T	Donor hysterectomy; recipient uterus allograft transplantation from cadaver or living donor

  a. 57155

  b. 58999

  c. 0664T

  d. 0667T

50. The physician orders and administers 600 mg of IV levofloxacin. How many units of code J1956 would be billed?

J1956	Injection, levofloxacin, 250 mg

  a. 1

  b. 2

  c. 3

  d. 4

51. Drs. Blank and Null are in the same cardiovascular practice. Dr. Blank is a cardiologist and Dr. Null is a cardiovascular surgeon. Dr. Blank has been seeing this Medicare patient for several years and now sends the patient to Dr. Null for consideration of a CABG procedure. What series of codes would Dr. Null use to code the services provided to this patient?

  a. Office or Other Outpatient Consultations, 99241–99245

  b. Inpatient Consultations, 99251–99255

  c. Office or Other Outpatient Services, New Patient, 99202–99205

  d. Office or Other Outpatient Services, Established Patient, 99211–99215

52. The coding professional notes that the physician has prescribed levothyroxine (Synthroid) for the patient. The coding professional might find which of the following on the patient's problem list?

  a. Acromegaly

  b. Hypothyroidism

  c. Dwarfism

  d. Cushing's disease

53. The clinical statement, "sections contain oral epithelium with underlying glandular tissue that has both serous and acinar cells" would be documented on which record form?

    a. Physical examination

    b. Operative report

    c. Pathology report

    d. Discharge summary

54. Chronic Care Management (CCM) may be provided by:

    a. Physicians

    b. Physician assistants

    c. Nurse practitioners

    d. All of the above

55. Which of the following is *not* considered an authoritative source by the CMS?

    a. American Hospital Association Coding Clinic for ICD-10-CM and ICD-10-PCS

    b. CPT Assistant

    c. American Hospital Association Coding Clinic for HCPCS

    d. ICD-10-CM and ICD-10-PCS Coding Handbook 2022 by AHA

Domain 4 *Compliance*

56. Which of the following would require a physician query regarding proper clinical documentation?

    a. The diagnoses given do not match word-for-word the title of the ICD-10-CM code.

    b. A diagnosis is given without supporting clinical documentation.

    c. The social history does not contain information about smoking or drinking habits.

    d. The chief complaint does not match the final diagnosis.

57. Under which of the following situations would it not be appropriate to query the physician?

    a. There is conflicting documentation in the record

    b. There is documentation on a procedure that is not supported by the diagnoses

    c. When a diagnosis of sepsis is not supported by blood work results

    d. When there is incomplete or illegible documentation

58. Queries are appropriate for documentation that is not legible, complete, clear, consistent, precise, reliable, or timely. Documentation that thoroughly describes what is occurring with the patient is considered to be:

    a. Consistent

    b. Clear

    c. Reliable

    d. Complete

59. When coding a colonoscopy with endoscopic removal of a tumor or polyp, what type of documentation would indicate ablation?

    a. Use of hot biopsy forceps or bipolar cautery

    b. Use of a snare followed by cauterization of the stump

    c. Use of a Nd:YAG laser

    d. Use of a Maloney dilator

60. When coding excision of a skin lesion, when should a separate code for wound repair be assigned?

    a. Wound repair is always coded separately from excision of a skin lesion.

    b. Excision of a skin lesion and wound repair should be coded separately when the repair is intermediate.

    c. Excision of a skin lesion and wound repair should be coded separately when there is repair by adjacent tissue transfer.

    d. Excision of a skin lesion and wound repair should be coded separately when tissue adhesive is used.

61. The coding professional is reviewing an operative report for wound debridement. In order to accurately assign a code for debridement, what information must be abstracted from the report?

    a. Method of biopsy

    b. Depth of tissue removed

    c. Type of repair performed

    d. Pathology results

62. Coding policies and procedures in any HIM Coding Compliance Manual should include all the following components *except*:

    a. AHIMA Code of Ethics

    b. Official Coding Guidelines

    c. AHIMA Standards of Ethical Coding

    d. Bylaws and Regulations of the Medical Staff

63. During an outpatient visit the attending physician did *not* define a problem at the conclusion of an emergency department (ED) visit. The coding professional should:

    a. Assign a code from the list of conditions in the history that occurred in the past.

    b. Assign a code for the reason for the last visit to the ED.

    c. Assign codes for abnormal laboratory findings.

    d. Assign a code for the chief complaint as the reason for the visit.

64. The specific legislation that provides for criminal penalties for healthcare professionals who knowingly and willfully attempt to defraud any of the healthcare benefit programs and further stipulates that physicians or other providers are accountable for information they know or should know is the:

    a. Federal False Claims Act

    b. Health Insurance Portability and Accountability Act

    c. Operation Restore Trust

    d. Balanced Budget Act of 1997

65. A patient is tested for COVID-19 and the test comes back negative. The patient was at a family gathering with a cousin who was later diagnosed with COVID-19. The physician documents pneumonia and influenza in the health record. What diagnosis codes are reported for this encounter?

    a. J11.00, J18.9, Z20.822

    b. J11.00, Z20.822

    c. J11.00, J18.9, U07.1

    d. J18.8, Z20.822

66. The patient is admitted with pneumonia due to COVID-19, which progresses to viral sepsis on day 3. What diagnosis codes are reported for this admission?

    a. U07.1, J12.89

    b. A41.89, J12.89, Z20.822

    c. U07.1, A41.89, J12.89

    d. A41.89, J12.89

67. The coding supervisor is auditing the coding of her newest staff member. In this particular case, the physician removed a skin lesion from the arm that was 3.0 cm by 2.0 cm. The operative and pathology reports also state that the physician took 1.0-cm margins. Final pathology results showed that the lesion was squamous cell carcinoma. The coding professional in training assigned code 11403. What feedback would the manager provide in the case?

    a. The manager would congratulate the trainee for excellent coding.

    b. The manager would explain that code 11406 should have been assigned.

    c. The manager would explain that code 11603 should have been assigned.

    d. The manager would explain that code 11606 should have been assigned.

68. An outside consultant has been retained to perform a coding audit for an orthopedist. He is reviewing an operative report for a patient who came in for a diagnostic arthroscopy of the elbow. The operative statement provided by the physician at the top of the report reads, "Diagnostic arthroscopy of the elbow." However, as he reviews the report, he sees that the physician describes the performance of a limited debridement during the course of the procedure. The case has been coded as: 29830, 29837. How would the consultant code this case?

    a. The consultant would code the case the same as the coding professional.

    b. The consultant would code only the diagnostic arthroscopy, 29830.

    c. The consultant would code only the arthroscopy with limited debridement, 29837.

    d. The consultant would code an arthroscopy with extensive debridement, 29838.

69. Which of the following statements would be an example of documentation that would meet the "Assessment" portion of the MEAT documentation review strategy:

    a. Lipid profile ordered

    b. A1c results reviewed with the patient

    c. Decreased sensation of BLE by monofilament test

    d. Advised on risks; smoking cessation counseling

70. CMS Hierarchical Condition Categories (HCC) models use data to:

    a. Predict long-term prognosis for individual patients

    b. Predict estimated future costs for individual patients

    c. Analyze treatment options for individual patients

    d. Predict mortality rates for trauma-related conditions

71. Under HIPAA's Privacy and Security Rules, which one of the following is *not* considered a covered entity?

    a. Healthcare providers

    b. Healthcare clearinghouse

    c. Life insurance company

    d. Health plan

72. Upon reviewing her record, Sally finds out that her physician stated in the discharge summary that she exhibited symptoms of extreme paranoia. Sally does not feel this statement is accurate and requests to amend her record. Which of the following would be a valid reason for Sally's physician to deny her request for amendment?

    a. Sally's physician feels the statement was accurate at the time.

    b. It is inappropriate to amend entries related to mental health.

    c. The request to amend the record was made greater than seven days postdischarge.

    d. Accepting the amendment may lessen the physician's reimbursement.

73. In which instance would informed consent *not* be required?

    a. The patient has a personal representative

    b. The patient is a minor

    c. At the physician's discretion

    d. In a medical emergency

74. Records maintained by a covered entity that are used to make decisions about an individual best describes:

    a. Business records

    b. Legal health records

    c. Limited data set

    d. Designated record set

75. A patient covered by Medicare is admitted on the evening of 1-14-2021. The attending physician completes the Initial Hospital Service while rounding the next day and submits the following codes to describe the service. What education should take place regarding this claim?

Date	CPT Code	ICD-10-CM Code
1-15-2021	99223, Initial hospital care, per day, for the evaluation and management of a patient, which requires these 3 key components: a comprehensive history; a comprehensive examination; and medical decision making of high complexity	S72.001A Fracture of unspecified part of neck of right femur, initial encounter for closed fracture

a. Level 3 initial hospital service codes are frequently the subject of government audits.

b. The ICD-10-CM code does not appear specific.

c. Modifier AI, Principal physician of record, was not assigned.

d. The date of service is incorrect.

76. An audit of orthopedic records indicates that the coding professionals consistently code application of casts or strapping (codes 29000–29584) after the orthopedic surgeons perform reductions of open fractures. As coding supervisor, what type of education would you give them on the use of codes 29000–29584?

   a. These codes are used only when the cast or strapping is an initial service without restorative treatment.

   b. These codes may be used with reductions of closed fractures only.

   c. These codes should only be used in the emergency department for restorative use.

   d. These codes may only be used by nonphysician providers.

77. In relation to Practice Expense in the RBRVS, which of the following is considered a nonfacility?

   a. Emergency department

   b. Skilled nursing facility

   c. Ambulatory surgical center

   d. Physician's office

78.

HCPCS CODE	Description	Work RVU	Non-facility PE	Facility PE	MP RVU
52317	Litholapaxy: crushing or fragmentation of calculus by any means in bladder and removal of fragments; simple or small (less than 2.5 cm)	6.71	17.48	2.55	.78

Locality Name	2020 PW GPCI	2020 PE GPCI	2020 MP GPCI
SAN DIEGO-CARLSBAD	1.032	1.130	0.607

Conversion Factor for 20XX: $36.88

How much would a physician be reimbursed in total by CMS and the patient for removing a bladder stone in the emergency room (the patient requested his own physician) in San Diego?

   a. $1,014.38

   b. $811.50

   c. $379.11

   d. $303.28

79. Services in a physician's office may be provided by a nonphysician provider when they are an incidental component of a physician's treatment. The physician must be actively involved in the care of the patient and supervise the nonphysician provider. This is called:

    a. Incident to billing

    b. Assistant to billing

    c. Assignment billing

    d. Integral to care billing

80. Which of the following nonphysician providers cannot bill for Medicare services under the Medicare Fee Schedule?

    a. Audiologists

    b. Midwives

    c. Registered nurses

    d. Psychologists

81. Which of the following is considered a nonfacility according to CMS?

    a. Urgent care facility

    b. Inpatient hospital

    c. On campus-outpatient hospital

    d. Off campus-outpatient hospital

82. Which of the following would be considered a leading query?

    a. Based on your clinical judgment, can you provide a diagnosis that represents the clinical indicators of pneumonia, WBC 14,000, respiratory rate 24, heart rate 20, hypotension, and altered mental status?

    b. The patient has elevated WBCs, tachycardia, and is given an IV antibiotic for *Pseudomonas* cultured from the blood. Are you treating for sepsis?

    c. Your impression in the H&P indicated that the patient has chronic congestive heart failure with an ejection fraction of 25 percent. Can the chronic heart failure be further specified?

    d. There is documentation of "angina" along with evidence of evaluation and treatment of the angina in the health record. Please document the underlying cause and type of angina, if known.

83. Dr. Duval is an orthopedic surgeon and a member of a large physician practice in Northeast New York. He has privileges at the Wharton General Hospital. He admits approximately 10 patients per month for hip replacement surgery. For these inpatients, his office staff will utilize what code set to bill for the hip replacement surgery?

    a. CPT

    b. HCPCS Level II

    c. ICD-10-PCS

    d. ICD-10-CM

84. Most facilities use to identify claim errors prior to claims submission?

    a. Manual review

    b. Coding professionals

    c. Compliance auditors

    d. Editing software

85. Which of the following adjudication outcomes results in a partial claim and error lines may be corrected and resubmitted?

    a. Deny

    b. Reject

    c. Suspend

    d. Hold

86. Which of the following compliance documents outlines the day-to-day operation rules for administering the CMS programs?

    a. Medicare Claims Processing Manual

    b. CMS Program transmittals

    c. National Correct Coding Initiative

    d. National Coverage Determinations

Domain 5   *Revenue Cycle*

87. Medicare's allowed fee for an in-office procedure is $200. Dr. Smith is a PAR physician, and Dr. Jones is a nonPAR physician who does not accept assignment. How much will Dr. Smith and Dr. Jones, respectively, receive from CMS?

    a. $160, $152

    b. $200, $152

    c. $160, $0

    d. $200, $0

88. Medicare's allowed fee for an in-office procedure is $200. Dr. Smith is a PAR physician, and Dr. Jones is a nonPAR physician who does not accept assignment. How much will Dr. Smith and Dr. Jones receive, respectively, in total for this procedure?

    a. $200, $200

    b. $160, $152

    c. $200, $218.50

    d. $200, $230

89. In the healthcare industry, what is the term for the written report that insurers use to notify the policyholder about the extent of payments made on a claim?

    a. Explanation of Benefits

    b. Summary of Benefits and Coverage

    c. Remittance Advice

    d. Medicare Explanation of Benefits

90. The _____ is a statement sent to the provider that explains the payments made by the third-party payers.

    a. Remittance Advice

    b. Advance Beneficiary Notice

    c. Attestation statement

    d. Explanation of Benefits

91. In RBRVS, this is an across-the-board national multiplier that is determined by CMS each year. It is the dollar amount that converts the relative value units into a payment amount:

    a. Geographic practice cost indices

    b. Pass-through payment

    c. Payment indicator

    d. Conversion factor

92. Which of the relative value units considers the costs of delivering healthcare services such as overhead, salaries of workers, and equipment?

    a. Work value

    b. Professional liability insurance

    c. Malpractice value

    d. Practice expense

93. This information is published by the area Medicare Administrative Contractors (MACs) to describe under what circumstances and within what time periods Medicare will cover a service. The ICD-10-CM and CPT/HCPCS codes are listed in the memoranda.

    a. Local Coverage Determination

    b. National Coverage Determination

    c. CMS

    d. Recovery Audit Contractors

94. Which of the following refers to the determination that a service is reasonable and necessary for the related diagnosis or treatment of illness or injury?

    a. Policy coverage

    b. Medical necessity

    c. Precertification

    d. Statutorily included

95. The physician has ordered an esophagogastroduodenoscopy (43235) for his patient. Which of the following ICD-10-CM codes would most likely justify the medical necessity of the examination?

    a. K28.3, Acute gastrojejunal ulcer without hemorrhage or perforation

    b. K26.3, Acute duodenal ulcer without hemorrhage or perforation

    c. K63.5, Polyp of colon

    d. J02.9, Acute pharyngitis, unspecified

96. A measure that assesses the ability to comply with billing edits is the:

    a. Denial rate

    b. Clean claim rate

    c. PEPPER rate

    d. Capture rate

97. The clinical documentation integrity (CDI) performance measure that indicates the number of times a physician responds to a CDI intervention divided by the number of CDI interventions issued is the:

    a. Physician response time rate

    b. Physician agreement with CDI specialist rate

    c. Physician response to CDI specialist rate

    d. Physician clarification rate

Multiple Choice Exam 1 Answers

1.	26.	51.	76.
2.	27.	52.	77.
3.	28.	53.	78.
4.	29.	54.	79.
5.	30.	55.	80.
6.	31.	56.	81.
7.	32.	57.	82.
8.	33.	58.	83.
9.	34.	59.	84.
10.	35.	60.	85.
11.	36.	61.	86.
12.	37.	62.	87.
13.	38.	63.	88.
14.	39.	64.	89.
15.	40.	65.	90.
16.	41.	66.	91.
17.	42.	67.	92.
18.	43.	68.	93.
19.	44.	69.	94.
20.	45.	70.	95.
21.	46.	71.	96.
22.	47.	72.	97.
23.	48.	73.	
24.	49.	74.	
25.	50.	75.	

EXAM 1 MEDICAL SCENARIOS

EXAM 1—SCENARIO 1

PICU PROGRESS NOTE

CHIEF COMPLAINT: Wheezing

HISTORY OF PRESENT ILLNESS: The patient is a 25-month-old male, transported here yesterday from the community hospital with a history of acute onset of respiratory distress and desaturation on room air. Clinical picture is initially consistent with first episode of wheezing. His respiratory distress has responded to Albuterol, Atrovent, Solu-Medrol, and Magnesium sulfate. However, he has persistent elevated anion gap that is not well explained.

OVERNIGHT EVENTS: The patient was initially treated with continuous albuterol at 10 mg/hr, Atrovent q 6 hours, Solu-Medrol × 6 hours, and he was given one dose of Magnesium sulfate IV for continued respiratory distress, with resulting decrease in tachypnea and improvement in wheezing. However, he showed a persistent metabolic acidosis with an elevated anion gap. Given that metabolic acidosis did not improve after aggressive fluid rehydration, and the anion gap was elevated, a search was carried out for possible etiologies. His initial serum glucose prior to initiation of steroid therapy was 178, and he did begin spilling ketones and glucose in his urine. We, therefore, elected to treat for possible diabetic ketoacidosis. His hyperglycemia rapidly resolved on Insulin 0.05 units/kg/hour and aggressive fluid and electrolyte replacement. He was quiet from a neurologic standpoint overnight, responding with appropriate distress to multiple blood draws and verbally interacting with parents. On further history, there is a family history of diabetes type 2 in grandmother. There is no antecedent polyuria or polydipsia. No weight loss. He had been completely well until 3 days prior to admission when he developed URI symptoms, which developed into acute respiratory distress yesterday, necessitating ED visit to outside hospital and subsequent transfer here.

PHYSICAL EXAMINATION

VITAL SIGNS:

    TEMPERATURE: 37.4

    HEART RATE: 147–199

    MBP: 60–95, R: 28–52

    OXYGEN SATURATION: 96–100%

    INPUT: 1,087

    OUTPUT: 853

GENERAL: Alert, says "No" or "Okay," appears more tired than yesterday's exam on admission, somewhat pale

HEENT: NCAT, TM's mildly red and partially wax impacted, no rhinorrhea, neck supple, no LAD

CARDIOVASCULAR: Tachycardia, regular sinus rhythm, no m/r/g

PULMONARY: Tachypnea, bilateral expiratory wheeze and prolonged expiratory phase, retractions

EXAM 1—SCENARIO 1 (*continued*)

ABDOMEN: Soft, ND/NT, 1BS, no masses or HSM

EXTREMITIES: WWP, symmetrical movements, CFT, 2 sec

NEURO: Somewhat more tired appearing than yesterday but still responds "Okay" to questions, symmetric movements UE and LE b/l, normal muscle bulk and tone, good strength when fighting blood draw today, EOMI, PERRL at 3 mm

LABS: Serum ketones 10 (elevated), urine glucose 250–800

CXR: Hyperinflation, PBT, no infiltrate

ASSESSMENT: Previously healthy 25-month-old boy with history of rapid onset of acute respiratory distress and wheezing. His pulmonary clinical picture is consistent with first-time reactive airway disease exacerbation with good response to typical asthma meds. However, he has persistent elevated anion gap acidosis and treatment for diabetic ketoacidosis is just beginning. Is on step 1 of new diabetes clinical pathway.

PLAN:

1. Diabetes mellitus, type 1, new onset. Follow clinical pathway, advancing diet to clears and assess tolerance. Follow I/Os. Get chem.–8 BID and CBC with lytes q 6 hours. Parents to step 1 education this afternoon.

2. Reactive airway disease, still with tachycardia and slightly tachypneic. Continue to observe as ketoacidosis resolves. Continue albuterol q 4 hrs prn. Transitioned from Solu-Medrol to Prednisone 2 mg/kg/day and will continue for total of 5-day course. Discontinue Atrovent. Repeat CXR prn for increasing respiratory distress.

3. Social work consult. Patient and parents are from out of state and visiting grandparents here. Mom in particular is quite worried about patient and his ability to complete travel plans to return home. Social work to assist with airline changes.

HISTORY: Detailed

EXAMINATION: Comprehensive

MEDICAL DECISION-MAKING: Moderate

Enter two diagnosis codes and one procedure code.

DX1

DX2

PR1

EXAM 1—SCENARIO 2

DATE OF EMERGENCY DEPARTMENT VISIT: 07/24/XX

CHIEF COMPLAINT: Right-sided chest pain

HISTORY OF PRESENT ILLNESS: The patient is a 47-year-old female who reports the onset of severe, sharp pain on her right side after an extended bout of coughing this afternoon. She reports the pain becoming acutely worse at approximately 5:30 p.m., again after another round of coughing. The patient is asthmatic and only in fair control. This last round of coughing resulted in post-tussive emesis. She reports that she is not short of breath but is breathing shallowly to avoid increasing the pain. There is no left-sided chest pain or pressure. She describes this pain as far different than any asthma-related pain. She tried her albuterol inhaler for the cough, but this had no relief of the pain. The pain is worse with deep inspiration and with movement of the chest. Other than the initial coughing episodes, there has been no focal trauma or direct injury to the area. She does report that she just returned from vacation yesterday, after a 5-hour airplane flight. She has not experienced any lower extremity pain or edema and is not actually short of breath. She has no history of deep vein thrombosis or pulmonary embolism.

PAST MEDICAL HISTORY:

1. Asthma

2. Gastroesophageal reflux

3. Migraine headaches

PAST SURGICAL HISTORY: Tubal ligation and bone spur removal from left foot in the remote past.

MEDICATIONS: Albuterol inhaler, Claritin, Prilosec, Singular, and Verapamil for headache prevention

ALLERGIES: Codeine

FAMILY HISTORY: Significant for asthma in mother and COPD in maternal grandfather.

SOCIAL HISTORY: She denies tobacco, alcohol, or drug abuse. She is accompanied to the ED by her husband.

REVIEW OF SYSTEMS: As per HPI and additionally, she denies fever, chills, or nausea. There is no diffuse weakness and no recent URI. There is no chest pressure, tightness, or palpitations. No sputum production with cough. No abdominal pain or diarrhea. No tingling or numbness. There are no rashes. Does not report any depression.

PHYSICAL EXAM: 141/96, Pulse 81, Respirations 24, Temp 97.6. The patient is awake and fully oriented. However, there appears to be moderate to severe distress from pain described above. Pupils: ERRLA bilaterally. The sclerae are white. Conjunctiva are pink. The oral mucosa is moist. The neck is supple with full ROM. No evidence of JVD. Lungs are clear to auscultation with breath sounds equal bilaterally. Heart is RRR, S1, S2 without murmur. Back is tender over the anterior or lower one third of the rib cage, including the lateral aspect of the left side of her chest. The sternum is nontender. There are no rashes. Abdomen is moderately obese but otherwise soft, nontender, and not distended with normal bowel sounds. Extremities are without cyanosis, clubbing, or edema. Homans sign is negative bilaterally. The calves are nontender. The radial and dorsalis pedis pulses are 2+ and equal bilaterally.

ED FINDINGS: A BMP revealed sodium of 137, potassium of 3.4, chloride 102, CO_2 27, BUN 11, creatinine 0.5, and glucose of 102. The D-dimer was normal at 0.24. Chest x-ray revealed mild elevation of the diaphragm on the right side but no evidence of pneumothorax. Otherwise, clear lung fields with a normal-appearing heart. CT of the chest to rule out PE revealed a little area of atelectasis with some fat and normal size lymph nodes in the hila, but no definitive evidence of PE.

ED COURSE: Initial suspicions were for pneumonia, pneumothorax, pulmonary embolism, costochondritis, or musculoskeletal pain. In light of her recent airplane flight, I felt that she was above a low risk for PE and obtained the above listed studies. The radiologist recommended the D-dimer, which returned normal.

EXAM 1—SCENARIO 2 (*continued*)

The patient's pain was controlled with IV Toradol and IV Morphine in the ED, and she had no evidence of tachycardia, tachypnea, or hypoxia on repeat evaluation. She felt comfortable with discharge and the diagnosis of costochondritis. She was given Vicodin for discomfort and will take ibuprofen 400 mg for anti-inflammatory, as tolerated by her GERD.

HISTORY: Comprehensive

EXAMINATION: Comprehensive

MEDICAL DECISION-MAKING: High

Enter four diagnosis codes and one procedure code.

DX1

DX2

DX3

DX4

PR1

EXAM 1—SCENARIO 3

PROCEDURE: Implantation of spinal cord stimulator lead under fluoroscopic guidance

DIAGNOSES: Chronic low back pain, lumbar radiculopathy, and multiple lumbar disc protrusions

The patient is well known to me, originally referred by Dr. X for management of chronic low back pain. The patient has tried multiple analgesics with partial relief. The patient has also had epidural steroid injections, which have given her temporary relief. The patient requested aggressive treatment, as the patient had a spinal cord stimulator trial done previously and was extremely happy with the degree of pain relief. The patient was also happy that she was able to sleep well and, she did not have to take her pain medications. The patient is very eager to get this permanent lead placement. It was decided to do a permanent spinal cord stimulator in lead as well as an implanted IPG. The patient also saw Dr. Y, who will be doing IPG implantation and the patient has also gone through the brochure as well as the video for the procedure. The patient understands the risks and benefits of the procedure. The patient understands its possible side effects, including headache from posterior puncture and also the possibility of weakness in the legs and epidural hematoma. The patient also understands that she should call me and the representative from Bionix as often as needed, if she has any side effects to call us, and to go to ER if needed. The patient also understands the restrictions advised to be followed sincerely.

PROCEDURE: Under monitored anesthesia care, the patient was positioned prone with arms extended upwards away from the surgical field. The patient's back was prepped aseptically. The patient was stable, spontaneously breathing, and communicating throughout the procedure. Radiographic C-arm was positioned directly over the thoracolumbar junction. Ll–L2 interspace was identified using fluoroscopy. Then 2 mL each of 1% lidocaine with 0.25 mL preservative free Marcaine was mixed and infiltrated using a 25-gauge needle to the inter laminar space. A #14-gauge Bionix epidural needle was then advanced toward the epidural space using paramedian approach by loss of resistance technique to air with 30- to 45-degree angle of entry. Epidural space was identified by lateral fluoroscopy continuously. On aspiration, no CSF or heme. No paresthesia at any point. The electrode was then advanced through the needle cephalad in epidural space directed to remain in the midline in the dorsal epidural space. The electrode was finally positioned at T8–T9 level. The patient appreciated appropriate paresthesia for stimulation covering her back and both the legs, especially the left lower extremity and back area. Further procedure was taken over by Dr. XX, who implanted the pulse generator and secured the lead as well as the pulse generator. In the recovery room, the patient complained of frontal headache, no nausea, or vomiting. The patient also complained of mild stiffness in the neck, which was partially reduced by Demerol 25 mg as well as 30 mg of Toradol. I again went over the patient with possible side effects of the procedure including posterior puncture headache, which may be the possible reason that she was having headache as well as neck stiffness. In detail, I explained to the patient the conservative management including analgesics, hydration, use of caffeine, and pain killers. I also explained the possibility of posterior puncture headache, treatment with blood patch. The patient will call me as needed and if the pain is significant will consider further aggressive treatment. The patient was discharged uneventfully. The patient has been prescribed Keflex. The patient has my number and the Bionix representative's telephone number to reach as needed.

Enter two diagnosis codes and one procedure code.

DX1

DX2

PR1

EXAM 1—SCENARIO 4

PREOPERATIVE DIAGNOSIS: Metastatic prostate cancer

POSTOPERATIVE DIAGNOSIS: Bilateral orchiectomy

PROCEDURE PERFORMED: Bilateral orchiectomy

INDICATIONS: This 71-year-old white male developed leg swelling, and a CT scan revealed retroperitoneal lymphadenopathy. Biopsy of these lymph nodes was positive for adenocarcinoma, PSA positive, suggesting prostate cancer. His PSA was 105 nanograms.

The options of treatment were discussed with the patient. He was advised to have bilateral orchiectomy. He has been started on Casodex. The patient agreed to surgery.

After satisfactory general anesthesia, the patient was prepped and draped in supine position. Incision was made in the median raphe of the scrotum. The testicular tunics were incised on the left side and the left testicle delivered from the wound. Spermatic cord was doubly clamped and excised. The spermatic cord was controlled with a proximal tie of #1 chromic catgut and a distal suture ligature of #1 chromic catgut. In similar fashion, the right testicle was removed. No complications were encountered. Wound was closed routinely in layers and sterile dressings applied, as well as a scrotal support. The patient was taken to the recovery room in good condition.

Enter two diagnosis codes and one procedure code.

DX1

DX2

PR1

EXAM 1—SCENARIO 5

PSYCHIATRY PROGRESS NOTE

DATE: 2/15/XX

LENGTH OF SERVICE: 55 minutes

LOCATION: Office

NOTES: The patient has continued to work on "Oceans of Emotions" workbook to help identify and understand her emotions better. Worked on short- and long-term goals—socially, academically, emotionally. She denies any difficulty with school with organization or concentration. She does endorse wanting more friends.

MSE: Alert, casually groomed wearing jeans and fleece; cooperative, good eye contact

SPEECH: Normal

THOUGHT PROCESS: Linear

THOUGHT CONTENT: Appropriate

MOOD: "Fine"

AFFECT: Somewhat anxious at times

INSIGHT AND JUDGMENT: Fair/good

ATTENTION: Fair

CHANGES TO MEDS SINCE LAST VISIT: None. No side effects reported. Good compliance.

CURRENT MEDS:

> Risperdal 1 mg TID
>
> Adderall XR 30 mg q a.m., Adderall 15 mg at 2 p.m.
>
> Celexa 5 mg q day
>
> Bactrim for acne

DIAGNOSES:

1. ADHD

2. Reactive adjustment disorder with anxiety

PLAN:

1. Continue current meds

2. Mother met with therapist for family therapy, patient to be scheduled in March

3. Insurance has approved up to 8 more visits

TREATMENT PLAN GOALS:

1. Decrease mood dysregulation

2. Decrease self-injurious behaviors

3. Decrease anxiety

4. Improve socialization

5. Improve self-esteem

6. Improve academic performance

Enter two diagnosis codes and one procedure code.

DX1

DX2

PR1

EXAM 1—SCENARIO 6

PROGRESS NOTE

DATE: 1/14/XX

LENGTH OF SERVICE: Approximately one and one-half hours

LOCATION: Physician's office

NOTES: The patient is receiving chemotherapy at this office for her previously diagnosed colorectal cancer.

TREATMENT: The patient receives 5-FU over 38 minutes, followed by Oxaliplatin for 42 minutes for chemotherapy and then receives a nonchemotherapy drug, Leucovorin for 5 minutes.

Enter two diagnosis codes and three procedure codes.

DX1

DX2

PR1

PR2

PR3

EXAM 1—SCENARIO 7

PREOPERATIVE DIAGNOSIS: Right upper lung tumor

POSTOPERATIVE DIAGNOSIS: Right upper lung tumor

OPERATION: Flexible bronchoscopy

ANESTHESIA: 2% xylocaine gel, xylocaine spray, and IV sedation

DESCRIPTION OF PROCEDURE: The patient was placed in the supine position. The right nostril was anesthetized with 2% xylocaine gel and the pharynx with xylocaine spray and 4% xylocaine liquid. After proper anesthesia the flexible bronchoscope was inserted into the right nostril without any difficulty. The pharynx and vocal cords looked normal. There were copious secretions over the cords and in the trachea; however, the trachea looks normal, the carina and the entire endobronchial tree, both the left side and the right side, look normal. Because of the lesions on the right upper lobe and possibly the right lower lobe superior segment noted on imaging, the bronchoscope was passed and then wedged in the right upper lobe where multiple endobronchial biopsies were taken. Also, biopsies from the right lower lobe superior segment were also taken. However, no lesions were seen. The old lumina looks open. The patient tolerated the procedure very well. Estimated blood loss was about 2 mL. The patient was taken to the recovery room in satisfactory condition, where a chest x-ray will be taken to rule out any pneumothorax.

Enter one diagnosis code and one procedure code.

DX1

PR1

EXAM 1—SCENARIO 8

ADMISSION DATE: 10/21/XX

DISCHARGE DATE: 10/24/XX

ADMISSION CHIEF COMPLAINT: Pneumonia

DISCHARGE DIAGNOSES: Pneumonia

PROCEDURES: Chest radiography

HOSPITAL COURSE: 7-week-old girl, ex 34-week preemie, presenting with 5 days of cough and runny nose and 1 day of fever to 100.8, vomiting ×4. Patient went to the local community hospital for a full sepsis workup and was transferred here for further treatment. Chest radiograph consistent with hyperinflation and lower respiratory infection. Patient was started on ampicillin and cefotaxime. She was also started on azithromycin given recent local pertussis epidemic. However, she did not clinically have signs or symptoms of pertussis during this admission. Her blood culture from the local hospital grew non-anthrax bacillus species on aerobic media, thought to potentially be a contaminant. Repeat blood culture after antibiotics before discharge showed no growth. Pertussis PCR negative.

Patient otherwise continued to stay afebrile throughout admission. She was monitored on IV antibiotics until discharge. She was discharged home when afebrile >24 hours, stable on RA and tolerating POs well. CBC one day prior to discharge was within normal limits. CSF culture is pending.

DISCHARGE STATUS: Recovered

DISCHARGE PLAN: I spent 45 minutes in education with the mother and grandmother, as well as treatment planning with primary care for follow-up after the CSF culture results return.

Enter one diagnosis code and one procedure code.

DX1

PR1

EXAM 2

Exam 2

For the following questions, choose the best answer. A blank answer sheet for these multiple-choice questions can be found on page 92.

Diagnosis Coding

1. The physician sees a patient in the hospital because an attempted therapeutic abortion resulted in a liveborn infant. In ICD-10-CM, how would the services provided to the mother be coded?

   a. Use the code for a complete or unspecified spontaneous abortion (O03.9).

   b. Use the code for the specific type of abortion along with a code from category Z37 (Outcome of delivery).

   c. Use the code for a missed abortion (O02.1) followed by code Z38.00 (Single liveborn infant, delivered vaginally).

   d. Use code Z33.2, (Encounter for elective termination of pregnancy) followed by Z37.0 (Single live birth).

2. How would the following be coded? Physician's office visit: Diagnosis of hypoglycemia in infant born to a diabetic mother.

   a. P70.0, Syndrome of infant of mother with gestational diabetes

   b. E08.649, Diabetes mellitus due to underlying condition with hypoglycemia without coma

   c. P70.1, Syndrome of infant of a diabetic mother

   d. E08.9, Diabetes mellitus due to underlying condition without complications

3. The patient is seen in his ophthalmologist's office and diagnosed with chronic angle-closure glaucoma, mild in the right eye and acute angle glaucoma in the left eye. Which diagnosis would the physician submit for these services?

H40.212	Acute angle-closure glaucoma, left eye
H40.2211	Chronic angle-closure glaucoma, right eye, mild stage
H40.20x1	Unspecified primary angle-closure glaucoma, mild stage
H40.1111	Primary open-angle glaucoma, right eye, mild stage

   a. H40.1111, H40.2211

   b. H40.212, H40.2211

   c. H40.212, H40.1111

   d. H40.2211, H40.20x1

4. The patient was seen in the outpatient wound care clinic for treatment of a decubitus ulcer of the sacrum. Upon examination, the physician listed the diagnosis as unstageable decubitus ulcer of the sacrum. How would this encounter be coded?

> | L89.100 | Pressure ulcer of unspecified part of back, unstageable |
> |---|---|
> | L89.109 | Pressure ulcer of unspecified part of back, unspecified stage |
> | L89.150 | Pressure ulcer of sacral region, unstageable |
> | L89.159 | Pressure ulcer of sacral region, unspecified stage |

  a. L89.100
  b. L89.159
  c. L89.150
  d. L89.109

5. The 20-year-old patient was seen in the emergency department with complaints that suggested a urinary tract infection to the physician. After a urine culture was done, the physician's diagnosis was confirmed as: Urinary tract infection due to Shiga toxin-producing *E. coli* O157. How would this diagnosis be coded?

> | N39.0 | Urinary tract infection, site not specified |
> |---|---|
> | P39.3 | Neonatal urinary tract infection |
> | B96.21 | Shiga toxin-producing Escherichia coli [E. coli] [STEC] O157 as the cause of diseases classified elsewhere |
> | B96.22 | Other specified Shiga toxin-producing Escherichia coli [E. coli] [STEC] as the cause of diseases classified elsewhere |
> | B96.23 | Unspecified Shiga toxin-producing Escherichia coli [E. coli] [STEC] as the cause of diseases classified elsewhere |

  a. N39.0, B96.21
  b. P39.3, B96.22
  c. N39.0, B96.23
  d. P39.3, B96.21

6. **In-office Chemotherapy Administration**

   The patient is a 73-year-old female who arrives today for her scheduled chemotherapy treatment. She is being treated for metastatic papillary serous cancer to lungs and brain.

   What diagnosis codes are reported for this encounter?

   a. C34.90, C79.31, C79.60
   b. C56.9, C78.00, C79.31, Z51.11
   c. C56.9, C78.00, C79.31
   d. Z51.11, C56.9, C78.00, C79.31

7. When the physician describes "deep full-thickness burns," he is referring to which degree of burn?

    a. First

    b. Second

    c. Third

    d. Fourth

8. A patient is seen in the emergency department with severe chest pain and was diagnosed with acute myocardial infarction of the anterolateral wall. He is given tissue plasminogen activator (tPA) and transferred within four hours to a cardiac specialty hospital. Which diagnosis would the physician submit for the hospital services at the specialty hospital?

> I21.09   ST elevation (STEMI) myocardial infarction involving other coronary artery of anterior wall
> I22.0   Subsequent ST elevation (STEMI) myocardial infarction of anterior wall
> Z92.82   Status post administration of tPA (rtPA) in a different facility within the last 24 hours prior to admission to current facility

    a. I21.09, Z92.82

    b. I22.0

    c. Z92.82

    d. I22.0, Z92.82

9. As it relates to the previous question, which diagnosis would the physician submit for the hospital services performed at the first hospital?

> I21.09   ST elevation (STEMI) myocardial infarction involving other coronary artery of anterior wall
> I22.0   Subsequent ST elevation (STEMI) myocardial infarction of anterior wall
> R07.89   Other chest pain
> Z92.82   Status post administration of tPA (rtPA) in a different facility within the last 24 hours prior to admission to current facility

    a. Z92.82

    b. I21.09

    c. I22.0

    d. R07.89

10. A Pap smear of the cervix cannot be interpreted because the sample was inadequate. What type of code should be assigned?

    a. Code that designates abnormal smear

    b. Code that designates satisfactory smear but lacking transformation zone

    c. Code for other abnormal Pap smear

    d. Code for unsatisfactory cytology smear

11. Nonhealing burns are coded as:

    a. Infected burns

    b. Chemical burns

    c. Acute burns

    d. Sunburn

12. The patient is admitted to the hospital for elective cholecystectomy for acute cholecystitis and cholelithiasis. Prior to the administration of anesthesia, the patient develops tachycardia and the surgery is cancelled. Which of the following would be used to report this encounter?

    a. K80.19, R00.0, Z53.09

    b. K80.00, R00.0, Z53.09

    c. K80.00, Z53.09

    d. K80.00, R00.0, Z53.01

13. The patient has been previously diagnosed with benign prostatic hypertrophy with urinary retention and presents for a TURP. The final diagnosis shows foci of adenocarcinoma. Which of the following codes would be used to report this encounter?

    a. D07.5, N40.1, R33.8

    b. C61, N40.0, R33.8

    c. C61, N40.1, R33.8

    d. D07.5, N40.1, R33.9

14. A female is admitted with postpartum perineum prolapse, which is secondary to second degree laceration that was sustained during a delivery 10 months ago. How would this diagnosis be coded?

N81.89	Other female genital prolapse
N81.9	Female genital prolapse, unspecified
O94	Sequelae of complications of pregnancy, childbirth, and the puerperium

    a. N81.89

    b. N81.89, O94

    c. O94

    d. N81.9, O94

15. The 71-year-old patient is seen in the office with secondary diabetes mellitus due to a previous partial pancreatectomy. Which diagnosis would the physician submit for the services?

E13.8	Other specified diabetes mellitus with unspecified complications
E13.9	Other specified diabetes mellitus without complications
E89.1	Postprocedural hypoinsulinemia
Z90.411	Acquired partial absence of pancreas

    a. E13.8, E89.1

    b. E89.1, Z90.411

    c. E89.1, E13.9, Z90.411

    d. E13.9, E89.1

16. Which is the correct way to code an encounter for a patient diagnosed with a basal cell carcinoma of the ear and external auditory canal?

C43.8	Malignant melanoma of overlapping sites of skin
C43.9	Malignant melanoma of skin, unspecified
C44.201	Unspecified malignant neoplasm of skin of unspecified ear and external auricular canal
C44.211	Basal cell carcinoma of skin of unspecified ear and external auricular canal

   a. C44.201
   b. C43.8
   c. C43.9
   d. C44.211

Domain 2 *Procedure Coding*

17. The patient presents for COVID-19 infectious agent testing. How is this procedure coded?
   a. 87633
   b. 87635
   c. 86769
   d. 86328

18. The patient presents for an initial insertion of a dual chamber pacemaker. How is this procedure coded?

33206	Insertion of new or replacement of permanent pacemaker with transvenous electrode(s); atrial
33208	atrial and ventricular
33216	Insertion of a single transvenous electrode, permanent pacemaker or implantable defibrillator
33217	Insertion of 2 transvenous electrodes, permanent pacemaker or implantable defibrillator

   a. 33206
   b. 33206, 33216
   c. 33208
   d. 33208, 33217

19. The physician completes a percutaneous transluminal coronary angioplasty on a patient with 90 percent acute blockage of two sites (proximal and mid) left anterior descending artery. A drug-eluting stent is used as each site. How is this service coded?
   a. 92920, 92928
   b. 92928
   c. 92928, 92929
   d. 92943

20. A new patient presents to the physician's office with complaints of migraines. The physician documents a medically appropriate history and physical exam. He documents that the patient has one undiagnosed new problem with an uncertain prognosis, orders a CT of the head, and prescribes medication for the patient's migraines. Which E/M code should be used to report the visit?

    a. 99202

    b. 99203

    c. 99204

    d. 99214

21. The patient is taken to the operating room by the neurosurgeon for repair of a depressed skull fracture following a motorcycle crash where he was an unhelmeted driver. Two large fragments of skull, one 7 cm and one 6 cm, have pierced the dura. The fragments are removed from the brain along with road contaminant, and the dura is repaired. How are the services of the neurosurgeon coded?

    a. 62000, Elevation of depressed skull fracture; simple, extradural

    b. 62005, Elevation of depressed skull fracture; compound or comminuted, extradural

    c. 62010, Elevation of depressed skull fracture; with repair of dura and/or debridement of brain

    d. 62141, Cranioplasty for skull defect; larger than 5 cm diameter

22. The coding professional is coding an arthrodesis of the interphalangeal joint, and the CPT Index has an entry that reads: Arthrodesis, Interphalangeal Joint 26860–26863. What action should the coding professional take?

    a. Code the first listed code in the series.

    b. Code the last listed code in the series.

    c. Look up codes 26860–26863 and code all the codes.

    d. Look up codes 26860–26863 and pick the best code.

23. The physician directly accesses an arteriovenous dialysis shunt using ultrasound guidance to visualize the puncture site. The shunt is completely imaged and evaluated for blockage. How is the procedure coded?

    a. 36901

    b. 37246

    c. 36215, 75710

    d. 36818, 76937

24. The patient presents with hallux rigidus of the right foot and undergoes the placement of an Integra flexible great toe implant following a cheilectomy. The arthritic joint is resected and implant is placed. How is this coded?

    a. 28289

    b. 28291

    c. 28292

    d. 28297

25. The physician injects the left facet joint nerves of L1 and L2 with a destructive agent, using fluoroscopic guidance. What is the correct code assignment for this case?

    a. 64635, 64636

    b. 64493, 64494

    c. 0216T, 0217T

    d. 64493, 64494, 77003

26. What information is necessary to assign the correct evaluation and management (E/M) code for preventive medicine services?

    a. The level of history and examination performed

    b. The counseling provided

    c. The risk factor reduction intervention

    d. The age of the patient

27. If a physician documents that he spent 10 minutes reviewing the patient's records, 20 minutes with the patient, and 5 minutes coordinating a referral, in what instance could we use this information to determine the level of E/M code?

    a. Preventive care visits

    b. Office or other outpatient visits

    c. Initial observation care

    d. Initial hospital care

28. When a patient is seen in the office and then admitted as an inpatient and discharged from the hospital all on the same calendar date, what series of codes should the coding professional use to code these services?

    a. Office and Other Outpatient Services and Hospital Discharge Services

    b. Observation or Inpatient Care Services (including Admission and Discharge Services)

    c. Office and Other Outpatient Services, Initial Hospital Care, and Hospital Discharge Services

    d. Initial Hospital Care and Hospital Discharge Services

29. A patient presents to the clinic for removal of her central venous access device (CVAD). The nurse practitioner documents a medically appropriate history and exam and medical decision-making of low complexity. She then removes the CVAD, bandaging the point of insertion. How should this encounter be coded?

    a. 99212

    b. 36589, 99212-25

    c. 99213

    d. 36589, 99213-25

30. A physician admits a patient to observation at 4:00 a.m. on June 15th. He documents a comprehensive history, a comprehensive examination, and medical decision-making of low complexity. The patient's condition improves throughout the day, and the physician elects to discharge the patient at 11:30 p.m. on June 15th. He spends 20 minutes with the patient explaining the patient's condition and plan for further workup. How would this case be coded?

    a. 99218, 99217

    b. 99219, 99217

    c. 99234

    d. 99235

31. A costovertebral approach is used for a posterolateral decompression of the spinal cord. The chest surgeon opens and closes the operative site and the neurosurgeon completes the decompression procedure. Which modifier is applied to the chest surgeon's services?

    a. -54, Surgical care only

    b. -62, Two surgeons

    c. -66, Surgical team

    d. -80, Assistant surgeon

32. When coding an E/M code, what modifier would be acceptable for use?

    a. -LT, Left side

    b. -32, Mandated services

    c. -51, Multiple procedures

    d. -59, Distinct procedural service

33. The patient lives in an assisted living facility that does not have nursing care. The caregiver calls the patient's physician to see the patient due to severe combativeness during meals. The physician provides an expanded problem-focused history and examination and uses moderate level medical decision-making. What code would the physician use to describe these services?

    a. 99232, Subsequent hospital care, per day, for the evaluation and management of a patient, which requires at least 2 of these 3 key components: an expanded problem focused interval history, an expanded problem focused examination, and medical decision making of moderate complexity

    b. 99308, Subsequent nursing facility care, per day, for the evaluation and management of a patient, which requires at least 2 of these 3 key components: an expanded problem focused interval history, an expanded problem focused examination, and examination and medical decision making of low complexity

    c. 99335, Domiciliary or rest home visit for the evaluation and management of an established patient, which requires at least 2 of these 3 key components: an expanded problem focused interval history, an expanded problem focused examination, and medical decision making of low complexity

    d. 99348, Home visit for the evaluation and management of an established patient, which requires at least 2 of these 3 key components: an expanded problem focused interval history, an expanded problem focused examination, and medical decision making of low complexity

34. The physician places a needle into the patient's back using intraoperative fluoroscopic guidance. The physician then injects local anesthetic and steroids into the epidural space bilaterally at the L4 and L5 level of the spine using a transforaminal approach. What is the correct procedure coding for this case?

64483	Injection(s), anesthetic agent(s) and/or steroid; transforaminal epidural, with imaging guidance (fluoroscopy or CT), lumbar or sacral, single level
64484	Injection(s), anesthetic agent(s) and/or steroid; transforaminal epidural, with imaging guidance (fluoroscopy or CT), lumbar or sacral, each additional level (List separately in addition to code for primary procedure)
64999	Unlisted procedure, nervous system
-50	Bilateral procedure

    a. 64999

    b. 64999-50

    c. 64483-50, 64484-50

    d. 64483-50, 64484, 64484

35. A patient is scheduled for an outpatient office visit on November 15. On November 14, the physician documents that she spent 15 minutes reviewing this longtime patient's record. On the day of the appointment, the physician documents a medically appropriate history and exam and that she spent 30 minutes with the patient and 5 minutes documenting in the EHR. Which E/M code should be reported?

    a. 99203

    b. 99204

    c. 99214

    d. 99215

36. A patient involved in a bicycle accident presents to the ER with multiple wounds on the left arm. The surgeon performs an intermediate repair of a 4.0 cm laceration on the forearm and a complex repair of a 2.0 cm laceration of the elbow. The shoulder wound is minor and does not require sutures. How should this procedure be coded?

    a. 12032, 13120-59

    b. 13120, 12032-59

    c. 12032-LT, 13120-LT

    d. 13120-LT, 12032-LT

37. The physician repairs a recurrent, reducible ventral hernia followed by implantation of mesh. How should this procedure be coded?

    a. 49565

    b. 49568

    c. 49565, 49568

    d. 49568, 49565

38. What code is assigned when four chest x-ray images are taken, two each from the anteroposterior (AP) and the lateral positions?

    a. 71045

    b. 71046

    c. 71047

    d. 71048

39. Which of the following is a true statement about the molecular pathology codes described in CPT?

    a. Tests in this section are quantitative unless otherwise noted.

    b. These tests are used to detect histocompatibility antigens.

    c. There are three tiers of test codes found in this section.

    d. Results for tests in this section are reported using the Bethesda system.

40. A 55-year-old male presents for a colonoscopy. The physician is unable to reach the splenic flexure due to poor preparation. What is the proper code assignment for the physician?

45330	Sigmoidoscopy, flexible; diagnostic, including collection of specimen(s) by brushing or washing, when performed (separate procedure)
45378	Colonoscopy, flexible; diagnostic, including collection of specimen(s) by brushing or washing, when performed (separate procedure)
-52	Reduced Services
-53	Discontinued Procedure
-74	Discontinued Out-Patient Hospital/Ambulatory Surgery Center (ASC) Procedure After Administration of Anesthesia

   a. 45330

   b. 45378-52

   c. 45378-53

   d. 45378-74

41. One part of a physician's office compliance plan is to respond appropriately to detected violations. Which of the following steps would be a first step of a corrective action plan if the office manager notices that the practice of unbundling is commonplace among the coding professionals?

   a. Issue oral warnings to all employees in the department.

   b. Refund overpayments from a third-party payer due to this practice.

   c. Post the new ICD-10-CM codes each year on the departmental bulletin board.

   d. Establish an open-door policy between the physician, the compliance officer, and the employees.

42. If during the course of an arthroscopic procedure, the physician must convert to an open procedure, which codes should be reported?

   a. Code(s) for the arthroscopic procedure only.

   b. Code(s) for the open procedure only.

   c. Code(s) for both the arthroscopic and open procedures.

   d. Code(s) for the arthroscopic procedure with a modifier to indicate increased procedural service.

43. The physician performs a herniorrhaphy to treat a reducible umbilical hernia on a three-year-old patient. How would this be coded?

49500	Repair initial inguinal hernia, age 6 months to younger than 5 years, with or without hydrocelectomy; reducible
49550	Repair initial femoral hernia, any age; reducible
49580	Repair umbilical hernia, younger than age 5 years; reducible
49585	Repair umbilical hernia, age 5 years or older; reducible

   a. 49500

   b. 49550

   c. 49580

   d. 49585

44. In his operative statement, the physician describes the procedure as "Cystoscopy with balloon dilation of a ureteral stricture." Upon reviewing the operative report, the coding professional notices that the physician mentions the placement of a temporary stent during the procedure. How should the coding professional code this operative report?

> | 52282 | Cystourethroscopy, with insertion of permanent urethral stent |
> |---|---|
> | 52332 | Cystourethroscopy, with insertion of indwelling ureteral stent (eg, Gibbons or double-J type) |
> | 52341 | Cystourethroscopy; with treatment of ureteral stricture (eg, balloon dilation, laser, electrocautery, and incision) |

    a. 52332

    b. 52341

    c. 52341, 52282

    d. 52341, 52332

45. The physician documents excision of a 2.0 cm condyloma of the penis. How would this be coded?

> | 11422 | Excision, benign lesion including margins, except skin tag (unless listed elsewhere), scalp, neck, hands, feet, genitalia; excised diameter 1.1 to 2.0 cm |
> |---|---|
> | 11622 | Excision, malignant lesion including margins, scalp, neck, hands, feet, genitalia; excised diameter 1.1 to 2 cm |
> | 54060 | Destruction of lesion(s), penis (eg, condyloma, papilloma, molluscum contagiosum, herpetic vesicle), simple; surgical excision |
> | -22 | Increased procedural services |

    a. 11422

    b. 11622

    c. 54060

    d. 54060-22

46. The physician performs a laparoscopic vaginal hysterectomy, including tubes and ovaries, on a 43-year-old female. The uterus weighs 280 g. How should this be coded?

> | 58291 | Vaginal hysterectomy, for uterus greater than 250 g; with removal of tube(s) and/or ovary(s) |
> |---|---|
> | 58554 | Laparoscopy, surgical, with vaginal hysterectomy, for uterus greater than 250 g; with removal of tube(s) and/or ovary(s) |
> | 58720 | Salpingo-oophorectomy, complete or partial, unilateral or bilateral (separate procedure) |

    a. 58291

    b. 58291, 58720

    c. 58554

    d. 58554, 58720

47. The physician performs a percutaneous transluminal coronary angioplasty in the left circumflex, followed by placement of a stent. He then performs a percutaneous transluminal coronary angioplasty with atherectomy in the left anterior descending coronary artery. How would this be coded?

92920	Percutaneous transluminal coronary angioplasty; single major coronary artery or branch
+92921	each additional branch of a major coronary artery (List separately in addition to code for primary procedure)
92924	Percutaneous transluminal coronary atherectomy, with coronary angioplasty when performed; single major coronary artery or branch
92928	Percutaneous transcatheter placement of intracoronary stent(s), with coronary angioplasty when performed; single major coronary artery or branch
+92929	each additional branch of a major coronary artery (List separately in addition to code for primary procedure)
-LC	Left circumflex coronary artery
-LD	Left anterior descending coronary artery

a. 92924-LD, 92920-LD, 92928-LC, 92920-LC

b. 92924-LD, 92921-LD, 92928-LC, 92921-LC

c. 92924-LD, 92929-LC

d. 92924-LD, 92928-LC

48. A physician is unable to complete the patient's mastectomy due to an adverse reaction to anesthesia. How should the physician report this procedure?

a. The physician is not allowed to report this procedure.

b. Submit the mastectomy code with modifier 52 for reduced services.

c. Submit the mastectomy code with modifier 53 for a discontinued procedure.

d. Submit the mastectomy code with modifier 74 for a discontinued outpatient procedure after administration of anesthesia.

Domain 3 *Research*

49. When a Medicare patient receives an IM injection of penicillin G benzathine, 100,000 units only, what is the appropriate code assignment?

96372	Therapeutic, prophylactic, or diagnostic injection (specify substance or drug); subcutaneous or intramuscular
96374	Therapeutic, prophylactic, or diagnostic injection (specify substance or drug); intravenous push, single or initial substance/drug
J0558	Injection, penicillin G benzathine, and penicillin G procaine, 100,000 units
J0561	Injection, penicillin G benzathine, 100,000 units

a. 96372

b. J0558

c. 96374

d. 96372, J0561

50. A Medicare patient with no symptoms or history of risk factors for colon cancer has a diagnostic endoscopy of the entire colon, from the rectum to the cecum and no issues were found. How is this coded?

    a. G0105, Colorectal cancer screening; colonoscopy on individual at high risk

    b. G0121, Colorectal cancer screening; colonoscopy on individual not meeting criteria for high risk

    c. 45330, Sigmoidoscopy, flexible; diagnostic, including collection of specimen(s) by brushing or washing, when performed (separate procedure)

    d. 45378, Colonoscopy, flexible; diagnostic, including collection of specimen(s) by brushing or washing, when performed (separate procedure)

51. Which one of the following is true regarding documenting queries to physicians?

    a. A verbal query between the physician and a clinical documentation specialist does not need to be recorded in the record.

    b. Queries should be destroyed after the physician answers the issue.

    c. Queries should be recorded as part of the permanent patient record or retained in other administrative records.

    d. Queries must only be retained in the patient record while the patient is hospitalized.

52. What is the best source of documentation to determine the size of a removed malignant lesion?

    a. Pathology report

    b. Postacute care unit record

    c. Operative report

    d. Physical examination

53. The physician performs an EGD followed by manual dilation. The coding professional is unsure if the code for the manual dilation can be reported with the code for the EGD. What should the coding professional reference to determine the official policy on reporting these codes together?

    a. National coverage determinations

    b. AHIMA website

    c. Current year's HCPCS annual update

    d. National Correct Coding Initiative (NCCI)

54. When coding excision of a lesion, from which report can the coding professional abstract the most accurate measurement?

    a. Operative report

    b. Pathology report

    c. Anesthesia record

    d. Nurses' notes

55. Which of the following is true regarding the guidelines for coding and reporting of diagnostic outpatient services?

    a. For patients receiving diagnostic services only during an encounter or a visit any documented diagnosis may be sequenced first for billing purposes.

    b. Without exception, the condition, problem, or reason for the encounter shown in the health record to be responsible for receiving the therapeutic services will be sequenced first for billing purposes for an outpatient encounter.

    c. For patients receiving preoperative evaluations only, sequence first a code from subcategory Z01.81, Encounter for pre-procedural examinations, to describe the pre

    d. For outpatient services, conditions documented as "probable," "possible," "suspected," "questionable," or "rule out" are to be coded as though they exist.

Domain 4 *Compliance*

56. The coding professional notes that the patient is taking prescribed Haldol. The final diagnoses on the progress notes include diabetes mellitus, acute pharyngitis, and malnutrition. What condition might the coding professional suspect the patient has and should query the physician?

    a. Insomnia

    b. Hypertension

    c. Schizophrenia

    d. Rheumatoid arthritis

57. Which of the following is not true about the query process?

    a. Queries must be in writing.

    b. Queries should be clear, concise, and nonleading.

    c. Queries should include pertinent findings and diagnoses documented in the health record.

    d. Queries should contain patient identifying information such as name and date of admission.

58. Which of the following is an example of a leading query?

    a. The patient has elevated WBCs, tachycardia, and is given an IV antibiotic for *Pseudomonas*. Are you treating for sepsis?

    b. Based on your clinical judgment, can you provide a diagnosis that represents the clinical indicators of elevated WBCs, tachycardia, and IV antibiotics for *Pseudomonas*?

    c. Do you agree with the pathology report specifying the "ovarian mass" as an "ovarian cancer"?

    d. Can the etiology of the patient's pneumonia be further specified?

59. The patient is seen by the physician and noted to have a chief complaint of shortness of breath. In the progress notes, the physician diagnoses asthma and recommends that the patient present to the emergency department of XYZ Hospital immediately. The physician further documents that the patient has severe wheezing and no obvious relief with bronchodilators. What should the coding professional do when preparing the bill?

    a. Code asthma.

    b. Code asthma with status asthmaticus.

    c. Code asthma with acute exacerbation.

    d. Query the physician for more detail about the asthma.

60. A patient comes into the physician's office for an IV infusion. In addition to the code for the infusion, the coding professional is considering adding an evaluation and management code with modifier 25. What documentation would be necessary to support the evaluation and management code?

    a. Documentation that meets the requirements of the documentation guidelines (history/exam/medical decision-making)

    b. A different diagnosis, and documentation that meets the requirements of the documentation guidelines (history/exam/medical decision-making)

    c. A different provider must document the evaluation and management service

    d. A separate evaluation and management code should never be reported on the same day as an infusion

61. When coding central venous access procedures, what type of documentation is needed for accurate code assignment?

    a. Single leads or dual leads?

    b. Vein transposition or direct anastomosis?

    c. Supervision and interpretation?

    d. Port or pump used?

62. Which of the following is *not* a risk area that the Office of the Inspector General has identified for physician practices?

    a. Billing for noncovered services as if they are covered

    b. Billing for a more expensive service than the one performed

    c. Developing, coordinating, and participating in coding training programs

    d. Coding and charging one or two middle levels of service codes exclusively

63. Which of the following is an example of abuse?

    a. Billing for services not provided

    b. Selling or sharing patients' Medicare numbers

    c. Performing occasional services considered by the carrier to be medically unnecessary

    d. Unbundling or exploding charges

64. The governmental agency that develops an annual work plan that delineates the specific target areas that will be monitored in a given year is the:

    a. Federal Bureau of Investigation

    b. Defense Criminal Investigative Service

    c. Office of the Inspector General

    d. US Attorneys' Offices

65. If a health record is being reviewed to ensure there are no missing physician signatures, the reviewer is likely performing:

    a. Quantitative analysis

    b. Qualitative analysis

    c. Coding audits

    d. Peer review

66. Which of the following is the *least* effective way to select an audit sample?

    a. Random sample of records for all physicians in a group

    b. All services provided on a randomly selected day

    c. Records selected by the physician for review

    d. All rejected claims during a specific time period

67. When reviewing activity reports, the manager notices that one coding professional consistently receives error messages when first attempting to submit codes for coronary artery bypass graft (CABG). She reviews the most recent record of a patient who underwent a CABG. The operative report states that two coronary arteries were bypassed by grafting the left internal mammary, and two sites were treated using grafts from the saphenous vein. The coding professional first attempted to submit 33518 followed by 33534. What must the manager explain to the coding professional to avoid this error in the future?

    a. In an example like this, only the venous grafts should be coded.

    b. In an example like this, only the arterial grafts should be coded.

    c. The venous grafts should be reported first, using the code 33511, not 33518.

    d. The arterial grafts (33534) should be reported first, since 33518 is an add-on code.

68. The coding auditor is reviewing evaluation and management codes. When reviewing the record of an ER patient, she finds that the physician documentation states that the physician provided 20 minutes of critical care in the emergency room. Additionally, he documented a detailed history, a detailed exam, and medical decision-making of high complexity. The encounter was coded as 99291. How would the auditor code this case?

    a. The same as the coding professional

    b. 99284

    c. 99285

    d. 99291, 99284-25

69. Which of the following conditions would not be included in the CMS-HCC model?

    a. Congestive heart failure

    b. Chronic obstructive pulmonary disease

    c. Acute renal failure

    d. Diabetes

70. Which of the following statements would be an example of documentation that would meet the *treatment* portion of the MEAT documentation review strategy?

    a. No complaints. Symptoms controlled on current meds.

    b. Managed by Dr. Smith.

    c. Relay wound measurement in exam.

    d. Pain controlled.

71. The patient has received copies of records from her health record that she requested earlier. In her request, she specifically asked for the discharge summary, the operative report, and the pathology report. The records that she received did not include the pathology report. The enclosed letter indicated the other document was not enclosed because of the Minimum Necessary Rule. What should the director tell the patient when she calls?

    a. The correct documents were sent. The patient can file a complaint with the hospital.

    b. The pathology report was not included in the designated record set so it was not sent.

    c. The Minimum Necessary Rule only allows access to dictated reports that have been transcribed.

    d. Everything she requested should have been sent since the patient is an exception to the Minimum Necessary Rule.

72. The patient has an appointment with a urologist for an initial visit. When must the patient be given the Notice of Privacy Practices?

    a. At the first visit

    b. When the patient receives his pre-appointment information

    c. Within two days after the first appointment

    d. At the second visit to the physician

73. A patient would like a copy of his health record sent to his aunt who is a physician, due to the fact that he is unable to explain his condition to her accurately. Which of the following statements in true according to the Privacy Rule?

    a. The physician can send a copy directly to the patient's aunt since she is a physician.

    b. The physician can send a copy directly to the patient's aunt if she pays the copy fee.

    c. The patient would need to sign a consent form in order for the physician to release the records to the patient's aunt.

    d. The patient would need to sign an authorization form in order for the physician to release the records to the patient's aunt.

74. Where might a patient find a description and examples of the covered entity's disclosures for treatment, payment, and healthcare operations?

    a. Authorization form

    b. Notice of privacy practices

    c. Consent for treatment

    d. Accounting of disclosures

75. Which of the following statements about surgical preparation codes 15002–15005 are true?

    a. Codes 15002–15005 are used when the wound will be healed by secondary intention.

    b. Codes 15002–15005 are the same as the debridement codes but are used with the skin graft codes.

    c. Codes 15002–15005 are to be used with autograft, flap or skin substitute graft.

    d. Codes 15002–15005 are not used with wounds to be treated by negative pressure wound therapy.

76. After reviewing this production report for June, what action should the coding manager take?

Production Report for Dr. Lyndon, Dermatology 6/1/XX to 6/30/XX				
CPT Code	Frequency	%	Charges	Payments
99212	156	46.2%	$5,772.00	$4,040.40
99213	147	43.6%	$7,350.00	$5,945.00
99214	10	2.9%	$730.00	$511.00
99215	24	7.1%	$2,712.00	$2,316.40
99243	56	65.1%	$7,000.00	$5,900.00
99244	27	31.3%	$4,050.00	$3,894.00
99245	3	3.4%	$600.00	$492.00

a. Educate Dr. Lyndon about the appropriate use of new patient codes.

b. Educate Dr. Lyndon on the correct percentages of consultation codes.

c. Determine why there were so few visits for the month.

d. Investigate why the charges were not paid in full.

77. Which of the following is true about the practice expense (PE) in the RBRVS?

a. The PE relative value unit is generally higher in the facility than for a nonfacility.

b. The selection for place of service is entirely up to the physician.

c. The PE is categorized as either facility or nonfacility.

d. There are three categories of PE costs according to the CMS.

78.

HCPCS CODE	Description	Work RVU	Nonfacility PE	Facility PE	MP RVU
28192	Removal of foreign body, foot; deep	4.78	8.24	3.75	.48

Locality Name	20XX PW GPCI	20XX PE GPCI	20XX MP GPCI
ALABAMA	1.000	0.889	0.707

What would be the total RVUs for a physician who removed a foreign body from the patient in an ambulatory surgical center in Alabama?

a. 8.453

b 9.01

c. 12.4446

d. 13.5

79. The physician assistant sees patient Jane Doe in the office; the sole physician is at the hospital doing surgery. How would the claim be submitted for this patient's visit?

a. The claim would be submitted using the physician's national provider identifier (NPI).

b. No claim would be submitted because the physician was unavailable.

c. The claim would be submitted using the physician assistant's NPI.

d. The charges submitted would be 50 percent of the normal charges due to the physician's absence.

80. A patient has an established diagnosis and has a chest x-ray taken. The patient sees the physician assistant to learn the results. The physician assistant reads the radiologist's report, makes appropriate notes in the health record, and discusses the findings with the patient. The physician is in the office during that time period. How would the claim be submitted for the patient's office visit?

    a. The claim would be submitted using the physician's national provider identifier (NPI).

    b. No claim would be submitted because the physician was unavailable.

    c. The claim would be submitted using the physician assistant's NPI.

    d. The charges submitted would be 50 percent of the normal charges due to the physician's absence.

81. Which of the following is not a benefit of single path coding?

    a. Duplicate processes are eliminated.

    b. Productivity is increased.

    c. Coding accuracy is enhanced.

    d. Coding professionals can focus on HCPCS coding for procedures.

82. Which of the following adjudication outcomes results in the facility having to appeal the payer's decision?

    a. Payment

    b. Reject

    c. Deny

    d. Hold

83. Which characteristic of quality documentation is defined as "the physician has fully addressed all concerns in the patient record; the entry has been signed and dated"?

    a. Legible

    b. Complete

    c. Consistent

    d. Timely

84. All of the following are examples of abuse except:

    a. Accidentally double billing for a service performed by the provider

    b. Knowingly billing for a service that the provider did not furnish

    c. Unbundling the components of a procedure rather than using one comprehensive code

    d. Misinterpreting coding guidance for a diagnosis code

85. Which of the following compliance documents is used by Medicare to communicate new policies and procedures for the various prospective payment systems?

    a. National coverage determinations

    b. Local coverage determinations

    c. CMS transmittals

    d. National Correct Coding Initiative

86. You are preparing an educational program related to mental, behavioral, and neurodevelopmental coding. Which of the following statements is true?

    a. Medical conditions due to substance abuse, use or dependence should be coded to F10.288, Alcohol dependence with other alcohol-induced disorder.

    b. Selection of the codes for mental health conditions "in remission" may be based on nonclinician assessments.

    c. The code for Munchausen's syndrome by proxy is assigned to the victim of abuse by their caregiver.

    d. The blood alcohol level does not need to be documented by the patient's provider in order for it to be coded.

Domain 5 *Revenue Cycle*

87. How often must an advanced beneficiary notice be signed when multiple instances of the same questionable service are provided?

    a. On an annual basis

    b. The first time the questionable service is provided

    c. On a monthly basis

    d. At the time each questionable service is provided

88. A physician's office can improve their copayment collections and increase revenue by using an electronic health record to assist them in:

    a. Benefits and eligibility checking

    b. Charge capture

    c. Scheduling

    d. Pharmacy benefits

89. A Medicare Summary Notice (MSN) is sent to the _____ to explain how payment was made on a claim.

    a. Physician performing the service

    b. Medicare beneficiary

    c. Hospital

    d. Non-Medicare beneficiary

90. The explanation of benefits (EOB) is sent to the:

    a. Third-party payer

    b. Provider

    c. Patient

    d. Hospital

91. In calculating the fee for a provider's service, each of the three relative value units is multiplied by the:

    a. National conversion factor

    b. Geographic practice cost indices

    c. Per diem amount set by CMS

    d. Usual and customary fees for the HCPCS code

92. Under RBRVS, all of the following are separate relative value units (RVUs) assigned for each CPT/HCPCS code, *except* for:

    a. Malpractice expense

    b. Physician's work

    c. Practice expense

    d. Geographic practice cost indices

93. What is the purpose of linking on a physician claim?

    a. Show how many times a service was provided

    b. Explain medical necessity of a procedure

    c. Group related surgical procedures together

    d. Show the day a procedure was performed

94. A coding manager reviewed the following information before the claim was submitted. What change would be required to ensure proper payment?

Patient Name	CPT Code	Description	ICD-10-CM Code	Description
John Doe	30300	Removal foreign body, intranasal; office type procedure	H44.701	Unspecified retained (old) intraocular foreign body, nonmagnetic, right eye

    a. A modifier is required on the CPT code.

    b. The diagnosis must be correctly linked to the procedure.

    c. The diagnosis code requires greater specificity.

    d. One or more additional CPT code(s) are required.

95. Which of the following is used to determine Medicare coverage by a Medicare Administrative Contractor, rather than nationwide, basis and assist providers with correct billing and claims processing?

    a. National Coverage Determinations

    b. Local Coverage Determinations

    c. Program Transmittals

    d. Correct Coding Initiative

96. A metric used to identify coding of secondary diagnoses is the:

    a. Denial rate

    b. Clean claim rate

    c. PEPPER rate

    d. Capture rate

97. Which of the following is considered a nonfacility setting in relation to the RBRVS (Resource-based Relative Value Scale)?

    a. Ambulatory surgical center

    b. Dialysis center

    c. Emergency department

    d. Outpatient hospital setting

Multiple Choice Exam 2 Answers

1.	26.	51.	76.
2.	27.	52.	77.
3.	28.	53.	78.
4.	29.	54.	79.
5.	30.	55.	80.
6.	31.	56.	81.
7.	32.	57.	82.
8.	33.	58.	83.
9.	34.	59.	84.
10.	35.	60.	85.
11.	36.	61.	86.
12.	37.	62.	87.
13.	38.	63.	88.
14.	39.	64.	89.
15.	40.	65.	90.
16.	41.	66.	91.
17.	42.	67.	92.
18.	43.	68.	93.
19.	44.	69.	94.
20.	45.	70.	95.
21.	46.	71.	96.
22.	47.	72.	97.
23.	48.	73.	
24.	49.	74.	
25.	50.	75.	

EXAM 2 MEDICAL SCENARIOS

EXAM 2—SCENARIO 1

PHYSICAL THERAPY EVALUATION

DATE: 1/28/XX

LENGTH OF SERVICE: 45 minutes

LOCATION: Office

NOTES: This patient is seen in Physical Therapy for an evaluation to initiate therapy. The patient is a 92-year-old male with a pattern of failing to follow through on any type of treatment plan. The patient is examined related to a left hip fracture that caused his last hospital admission. Type 2 Diabetes with diabetic neuropathy is evaluated as well as compromised skin of the left lower extremity in the area of a previous heel ulcer. The patient has borderline obesity affecting his mobility. A moderately complex treatment plan was developed and fully documented during this 45-minute visit.

Enter four diagnosis codes and one procedure code.

DX1

DX2

DX3

DX4

PR1

EXAM 2—SCENARIO 2

OFFICE VISIT

CHIEF COMPLAINT: Diarrhea and nausea

HISTORY OF PRESENT ILLNESS: This is a 70-year-old Caucasian male, established patient, who presents today to the office with complaints of diarrhea, and nausea present over the past 6 weeks that have increased gradually in frequency. Currently, he's having diarrhea 3 times a day. It's watery at times, sometimes soft. He thinks that things are worsening. The color of the stool is tan or brown. He has no black or tarry stools. He notes no bright red blood per rectum. He does admit to lethargy.

Upon questioning, he does admit to being on an antibiotic recently, approximately 6 weeks ago. Before his symptoms started, he had been put on Z-Pak for some sinus symptoms, and he did notice that his symptoms started after being on the Z-Pak.

He was started on Prilosec several weeks ago for some irritation due to Fosamax and he has been on Prilosec since then.

In addition, he relates today that he was scratched by some dogs and according to our chart, hasn't had a tetanus shot since 1998.

PAST MEDICAL HISTORY:

Numerous medical issues, in particular:

1. Cardiac issues

2. Hypertension

3. Hypercholesterolemia

CURRENT MEDICATIONS:

1. Aspirin

2. Calcium

3. Ticlid

4. Zocor

5. Prilosec

SOCIAL HISTORY: He denies alcohol or tobacco.

REVIEW OF SYSTEMS: Negative for chest pain or shortness of breath. He does admit to increased flatulence and abdominal pain, only after eating, which resolves after the flatulence resolves.

PHYSICAL EXAMINATION:

VITAL SIGNS:

> **BLOOD PRESSURE:** 120/54
>
> **PULSE:** 56
>
> **TEMPERATURE:** 98.1
>
> **WEIGHT:** 135

GENERAL: He is in no acute distress. Able to give a good history. He's alert and oriented without evidence of severe lethargy or fatigue.

EXAM 2—SCENARIO 2 (*continued*)

HEART: Regular rate and rhythm. No murmurs, gallops, or rubs or heaves.

LUNGS: Clear to auscultation

ABDOMEN: Soft and nontender. No organomegaly. Hyperactive bowel sounds. No skin changes.

EXTREMITIES: Without cyanosis, clubbing, or edema

SKIN: No abnormalities, except for several abrasions and excoriations on his anterior arms due to dogs scratching at him today.

ASSESSMENT AND PLAN:

1. I gave him a Td shot today. The abrasions are somewhat deep and have some debris. I cleansed the one on the right forearm and rebandaged it.

2. With regard to his significant diarrhea, I do want to rule out *C. difficile*, so will send off a stool for *C. difficile* blood count toxin. I will also send off a culture to rule out *Salmonella, Shigella*, or enteric *Campylobacter*, and I also asked him to stop the Prilosec right now to see if his symptoms improve off Prilosec as this may be an offending agent as well.

3. All questions were answered. He will return the stool sample in the morning.

HISTORY: Detailed

EXAMINATION: Detailed

MEDICAL DECISION-MAKING: Moderate level

TOTAL TIME SPENT WITH PATIENT: 35 minutes

Enter four diagnosis codes and three procedure codes.

DX1

DX2

DX3

DX4

PR1

PR2

PR3

EXAM 2—SCENARIO 3

DATE OF ADMISSION: 01/15/20XX

DATE OF CONSULTATION: 01/15/20XX

REQUESTED BY: Dr. Y

CHIEF COMPLAINT: Not feeling good and constipation

CONSULT SERVICE: Endocrinology

HISTORY OF PRESENT ILLNESS: The patient is a 4-year-old male who was taken to the emergency department by his parents because he had constipation, and he was subsequently admitted as an inpatient. He has had no stools for 5 days. He also began vomiting the morning of admission. He has had decreased food intake over the past 5 days. He has had polyuria and polydipsia for the past 2 months, also bedwetting for 1 to 2 months. He has had a 7-lb weight loss. He had not been complaining of abdominal pain, no complaints of blurred vision, no complaints of headache.

In the emergency department, by mom's report, he was given an enema. They also elected to do some labs. He was found to have a blood sugar level over 400 and a pH of 7.10. He was admitted to the pediatric intensive care unit.

PAST MEDICAL HISTORY: He was the product of a normal pregnancy. Birth weight 8 lb 10 oz. He has had no hospitalizations. He has no known drug allergies.

FAMILY HISTORY: Negative for type 1 diabetes. There is type 2 diabetes only in a maternal great-grandmother. There is a maternal grandmother with rheumatoid arthritis, thyroid conditions, cardiovascular disease (had CABG in mid-40s), and dyslipidemia. Mom is not aware of any issues regarding health on the maternal grandfather's side of the family, but admittedly does not know much about her father's history. His father is Filipino/Samoan ethnicity, knows of no diabetes in the family, and no major health conditions. The patient has a 2-year-old brother who is healthy. Mom is 35 weeks pregnant. She has had no gestational diabetes. Father had some cold symptoms, and the patient also developed cold symptoms in the past week.

SOCIAL HISTORY: The patient lives with his parents and sibling.

REVIEW OF SYMPTOMS: Negative for fever or fatigue. There has been a 5- to 7-lb weight loss as mentioned above. Nasal discharge as mentioned above, no complaints of sore throat, mild cough, no chest pain, decreased appetite, vomiting and constipation as mentioned above, polyuria, polydipsia, nocturia, no dysuria, no weakness, no headaches. Regarding mood changes, Mom has noted that he has seemed to have more behavioral issues upon eating sugar. Mom does believe his skin and lips to be dry for the past few weeks.

PHYSICAL EXAMINATION: The patient is an alert, smiling boy in no distress. Weight 25.1 kg, temperature 36.7, pulse 119, respiratory rate 18, blood pressure 99/79.

HEENT: Conjunctivae normal. Pupils reactive. Glimpses of his fundi normal. Oral mucosa moist. Breath not fruity in odor. No oropharyngeal exudate.

NECK: Supple with no thyroid enlargement

LUNGS: Clear, no wheezing

CARDIAC: Normal rhythm, no murmur

ABDOMEN: Soft, nontender, normal bowel sounds

EXAM 2—SCENARIO 3 *(continued)*

GENITALIA: He had normal prepubertal genitalia. Testes descended bilaterally.

SKIN: Notable for 2 small café-au-lait spots on his trunk, slightly doughy texture of his skin

NEUROLOGIC: Sensation was grossly intact. He had normal speech.

LABORATORY STUDIES: On admission, venous pH 7.10, blood glucose 449, sodium 144, potassium 4.3, chloride 110, CO_2 less than 5, BUN 7, creatinine 0.6, calcium 11.2, magnesium 2.2, phosphorus 4.2. CBC was remarkable for a white blood cell count of 13.5, 63 polyps, 22 lymphocytes, 10 monocytes, hematocrit 46.3. Hemoglobin A1c pending at the time of this dictation.

IMPRESSION: This is a 4-year-old patient with new-onset type 1 diabetes, presenting in severe diabetic ketoacidosis (DKA). His DKA is resolving. DKA management as per diabetes clinical pathway, he is currently on an insulin infusion at 0.1 units per kg/hour and D10 fluids. Blood glucose checked q2h, electrolytes q4h at present. He will be transitioned to subcutaneous insulin later in the day, starting at 1 unit per kg per day. In view of the family situation, with Mom's upcoming delivery, likely NPH and Humalog insulin will be a bit easier for this family. Diabetes education will begin today with diabetes nurse educator, and later in the week with a nutritionist and social worker.

Regarding constipation, we will continue to follow this. Also, of note is the fact that on his initial studies he had 2+ protein as well as ketonuria. Would recheck urinalysis later during his hospital stay. Patient to be transferred from unit and will be on the Endocrine Service.

HISTORY: Comprehensive

EXAMINATION: Comprehensive

MEDICAL DECISION-MAKING: High

Enter two diagnosis codes and one procedure code.

DX1

DX2

PR1

EXAM 2—SCENARIO 4

DATE OF PROCEDURE: 10/30/20XX

PREOPERATIVE DIAGNOSIS: Traumatic left quadriceps tendon rupture

POSTOPERATIVE DIAGNOSIS: Traumatic left quadriceps tendon rupture

PROCEDURE: Repair of left quadriceps tendon rupture

ANESTHESIA: Spinal

COMPLICATIONS: None

DRAINS: None

ESTIMATED BLOOD LOSS: 50 cc to 100 cc

PROCEDURE: The patient was brought to the operating room and after the instillation of a satisfactory spinal anesthesia, the left lower extremity was appropriately prepared and draped in the usual sterile fashion. A midline incision was made and centered over the patella and carried down to the quadriceps mechanism. Medial and lateral dissection was carried out to expose the retinaculum, which was torn approximately 2 cm laterally and medially. There was a direct avulsion of the quadriceps tendon off the patella with a small fleck of osteophytic bone. The quadriceps tendon was freshened. Also, the bony surface of the patella was debrided of soft tissue and hematoma and fibrous tissue. Once this was repaired, three holes, center, mid lateral, and mid medial were marked. Following this, a #5 Ethibond and #2 FiberWire were placed in the quadriceps mechanism both medially and laterally, beginning in the midportion with a Krackow suture. Following this, three drill holes were made longitudinally from superior to inferior through the patella and a suture passer was used to retrieve the ends of the suture. When these were secured, the quad tendon was brought down into the patellar bed. Following this, #2 Ethibond retinacular sutures were added from the superolateral and superomedial junction of the patella laterally and medially. These were then tightened. As they were tightened, the sutures in the patella were securely tightened as well. The retinacular sutures were then tightened. Supplemental 2-0 Vicryl anteriorly into the quad tendon and patellar soft tissue and retinaculum was then accomplished. This knee could be flexed to about 30 degrees before there was significant tension on this quadriceps tendon. Therefore, we will be holding him in extension. Following this, a thorough Waterpik irrigation was accomplished. The subcutaneous was closed with interrupted 2-0 Vicryl, and the skin closed with skin clips. A sterile dressing and a knee immobilizer were placed.

The patient was taken to the recovery room in satisfactory condition.

Enter one diagnosis code and one procedure code.

DX1

PR1

EXAM 2—SCENARIO 5

DATE OF OPERATION: 01/30/20XX

PREOPERATIVE DIAGNOSIS: Multiple myeloma with pending stem cell transplant

POSTOPERATIVE DIAGNOSIS: Multiple myeloma with pending stem cell transplant

PROCEDURE: Placement of tunneled central venous NeoStar catheter via the right internal jugular vein with ultrasound and fluoroscopic assistance.

ANESTHESIA: Local with MAC

ESTIMATED BLOOD LOSS: Minimal

FLUIDS: 750 mL of crystalloid

DRAINS: None

SPECIMENS: None

COMPLICATIONS: A male with a diagnosis of multiple myeloma. Stem cell transplantation is pending, and the patient is in need of a central venous catheter suitable for pheresis.

PROCEDURE: After obtaining informed consent, the patient was brought to the operating room and placed supine on the operating table. The skin of the anterior chest and neck was shaved, prepared, and draped in the standard sterile fashion. Using ultrasound guidance by Dr. X, a needle with syringe was advanced into the internal jugular vein with good blood return. A larger introducer needle was then advanced parallel to the previous needle under ultrasound guidance and placed into the right internal jugular vein with good blood return. A guidewire was advanced through the introducer needle under fluoroscopic guidance. The needle was then removed, leaving the guidewire in place. A 5-mm incision was made at the site of the wire exiting the skin with a #11 blade scalpel. It should be noted that the skin of the right neck was anesthetized with 1% lidocaine for analgesia. At this point, a suitable location in the right chest was chosen for the catheter exit site.

This area, as well as the subcutaneous tract, was anesthetized with 1% lidocaine. A 5-mm skin incision was made at the anticipated catheter exit site with a #11 blade scalpel. A tunneler device was then used to create the subcutaneous tunnel, bringing the tunneler in a cephalad fashion and out through the previous skin incision in the neck.

At this point, a dilator was passed over the guidewire under fluoroscopy to dilate the tract. This was done serially. An introducer peel-away catheter was threaded over the guidewire, and the guidewire was then removed. The previously tunneled NeoStar catheter was then advanced through the peel-away sheath under fluoroscopy. The sheath was removed, and the catheter had a good position in the cavoatrial junction. There was an acute angle in the catheter site as it exited the fascia of the neck. This was corrected by extending the skin incision and creating a nice curve in the catheter without kinks. Again, distal placement was confirmed at the cavoatrial junction under live fluoroscopy. The catheter withdrew blood and flushed easily at all three ports. One thousand units per cc of heparin flush were used to heplock the catheter. The catheter was secured to the skin of the right chest with a 4-0 Prolene suture. A 4-0 Vicryl was then used to reapproximate the skin of the neck incision. Dermabond was applied to the neck incision site, and sterile dressings were applied. The patient tolerated the procedure well and without any complications. A chest x-ray is pending in the recovery room to confirm adequate placement of the catheter and to rule out a pneumothorax.

Enter one diagnosis code and one procedure code.

DX1

PR1

EXAM 2—SCENARIO 6

OUTPATIENT HEMODIALYSIS CLINIC

DATE: 2/24/XX

LOCATION: Outpatient clinic

NOTES: The patient is being seen today for hemodialysis due to his long-standing diagnosis of end-stage renal failure. He presents today following evaluation by his personal physician for his first hemodialysis treatment.

Enter one diagnosis code and one procedure code.

DX1

PR1

EXAM 2—SCENARIO 7

DATE OF OPERATION: 01/05/20XX

PREOPERATIVE DIAGNOSIS: Congenital cataract of the right eye

POSTOPERATIVE DIAGNOSIS: Congenital cataract of the right eye

OPERATION: Cataract extraction with primary posterior capsulotomy and limited anterior vitrectomy with intraocular lens.

INDICATIONS: Patient with a congenital cataract of the right eye, needed to have surgical intervention to remove it, which was performed here today.

ANESTHESIA: General orotracheal anesthesia

ESTIMATED BLOOD LOSS: Negligible

COMPLICATIONS: None

SPECIMENS SENT TO PATHOLOGY: None

PROCEDURE IN DETAIL: The patient was brought back to the operating room, adequately premedicated, and intubated without complications. Directly after induction, the patient had pressures taken in both eyes and was found to have a pressure in the right eye of 16 and in the left eye of 17.

That was within 2 minutes of induction, error rate less than 5%.

Then keratometry readings were performed, three sets of two readings on each eye. On the right eye 44.5 × 46.25. Second reading is 44 × 46.25. The third reading is 44.5 × 46. In the left eye, 44.75 × 45, 44.25 × 45, and 43.75 × 45. Central corneal thickness for the right eye was 593 microns ± 1.5 microns and left eye 562 microns ±1.8 microns. Axial lengths were then measured using I3 ultrasound. For the right eye, the axial length was found to be 20.28 and the left eye 20.44. With the given K's and the axial lengths for the right eye, it was determined that for approximately 2 to 2.5 undercorrection, a 27.5 lens needed to be put in his eye and that was the one that was chosen.

Then the patient was prepared and draped in the usual sterile ophthalmic fashion after he received several mydriatic and cycloplegic drops. He also received one drop of Ciloxan to the right eye every 5 minutes for three drops and then one drop of flurbiprofen to the right eye every 5 minutes × 3. Once the patient was prepared and draped in the usual sterile ophthalmic fashion, a limited lateral peritomy was performed.

Hemostasis was achieved with bipolar cautery and then a keratome was used to enter the eye. Healon GV was placed in the eye to maintain anterior chamber formation.

A super-sharp blade was used to make a paracentesis at 6 o'clock. Then a cystotome was used to make a rent in the anterior capsule. A continuous curvilinear capsulorrhexis was attempted with a capsulorrhexis forceps. However, the cataract was such that it was anterior polar in nature and it was off center. It wasn't directly on the pupillary axis. That anterior polar protrusion made it so that continuing the continuous curvilinear capsulorrhexis was impossible, so a vitrector was placed in the eye. The lens was removed, including the cataract. Then Healon GV was used to inflate the eye again. A rent was made in the posterior capsule, and a limited anterior vitrectomy was performed through that rent. The incision was widened with a 3.2 short cut blade and then a 27.5 diopter SA60AT single piece intraocular lens was injected into the eye, serial number 829167.075, and the lens was rotated to be in place. It was found to be in good position.

The Healon was removed with aspiration of the vitrector. The incision was closed with a double armed 8-0 Vicryl suture, mattress fashion suturing of the incision. It was found to be water tight. Then the conjunctiva was closed with one interrupted 7-0 chromic gut suture. 2.5 cc of dexamethasone was injected over the incision and then 0.4 cc of Kefzol was injected in the inferonasal quadrant.

EXAM 2—SCENARIO 7 (*continued*)

Betadine, followed by TobraDex. A pressure patch, followed by a shield, was then placed on his eye and held in place with Tegaderm. The patient tolerated the procedure well. He was extubated in the operating room and taken to the recovery room in satisfactory condition.

Enter one diagnosis code and one procedure code.

DX1

PR1

EXAM 2—SCENARIO 8

DATE OF PROCEDURE: 11/21/20XX

PROCEDURE: 24-hour pH probe

INDICATIONS: The patient is a complicated teenager with type 1 diabetes who has had issues with delayed gastric emptying. She is a known diabetic and she does have GI reflux. She is here for full evaluation of that symptom complex and is accompanied by her mother, who has signed an informed consent.

The double-bore pH probe was placed nasally when the patient was under anesthesia. The overall Boix-Ochoa score was 24.5, with normal being less than 16.6. There was no reflux during the night when she was asleep with the exception of one very prolonged episode that lasted 26.3 minutes. The overall reflux score was 6.8% with normal being less than 5.1%.

It would be advisable for her to stay on the medication profile that she is already taking but I do not think she is a candidate for surgery.

Enter three diagnosis codes and one procedure code.

DX1

DX2

DX3

PR1

EXAM 3

For the following questions, choose the best answer. A blank answer sheet for these multiple-choice questions can be found on page 130.

Domain 1 *Diagnosis Coding*

1. In ICD-10-CM, which one of the following conditions is a mechanical complication of an internal implant, device, or graft?

   a. Scarring due to presence of breast implants

   b. Inflammation due to indwelling catheter

   c. Pain due to renal dialysis device

   d. Obstruction of heart valve prostheses

2. A female patient is seen in the physician's office because of pain in her right lower leg. The leg was red and swollen. The physician was concerned because the patient was postoperative and after a careful examination, rendered the final impression of: Postoperative cellulitis of right lower leg. How is this coded?

L03.115	Cellulitis of right lower limb
L03.119	Cellulitis of unspecified part of limb
T81.40XA	Infection following a procedure, unspecified, initial encounter

   a. T81.40XA

   b. L03.115

   c. T81.40XA, L03.119

   d. T81.40XA, L03.115

3. In ICD-10-CM, a young primigravida is defined as:

   a. Second or more pregnancy in a female less than 16 years old at time of delivery

   b. First pregnancy in a female less than 16 years old at time of delivery

   c. First delivery in a female less than 15 years old

   d. Second delivery in a female less than 15 years old

4. A female who is not currently pregnant but has a history of recurrent pregnancy loss is best described by which of the following code statements?

   a. N96, Recurrent pregnancy loss

   b. O26.2-, Pregnancy care for patient with recurrent pregnancy loss

   c. Z87.51, Personal history of pre-term labor

   d. Z87.59, Personal history of other complications of pregnancy, childbirth, and the puerperium

5. An elderly patient comes to the emergency department complaining of left upper arm pain. The physician orders an x-ray and questions the patient about a possible injury. The patient states she did not fall or hurt her arm in any way. It simply hurt when she woke up. After reviewing the x-ray report, the physician notices a fracture of the humerus. Considering other conditions that the patient has, his final diagnosis is pathological fracture of the humerus. How would this case be coded?

   a. M84.422A, Pathological fracture, left humerus, initial encounter for fracture

   b. M84.522A, Pathological fracture in neoplastic disease, left humerus, initial encounter for fracture

   c. M80.022A, Age-related osteoporosis with current pathological fracture, left humerus, initial encounter for fracture

   d. S42.302A, Unspecified fracture of shaft of humerus, left arm, initial encounter for closed fracture

6. The 26-year-old female diabetic patient is admitted with ketoacidosis. She recently had wisdom teeth removal with a subsequent abscess of the nearby tooth. This appears to be the source of the poorly controlled type 1 diabetes mellitus. The patient was rehydrated due to dehydration and was given IV antibiotics for the abscess. Which of the following codes would be reported?

   a. E11.65, K04.7, E86.0

   b. E10.10, E87.2, E10.65, K04.7, E86.0

   c. E10.10, E10.65, K04.7, E86.0

   d. E11.65, E87.2, K04.7, E86.0

7. Symptomatic HIV infection should be coded to which of the following codes?

   a. R75, Inconclusive laboratory evidence of human immunodeficiency virus [HIV]

   b. B20, Human immunodeficiency virus [HIV] disease

   c. Z72.51, High risk heterosexual behavior

   d. Z21, Asymptomatic human immunodeficiency virus [HIV] infection status

8. In ICD-10-CM, burns are classified in Category T31 according to the extent of body surface involved. What rule is involved in estimating this body surface?

   a. Code only any third-degree burns.

   b. Code burns as a late effect.

   c. Code according to the rule of nines.

   d. Code burns as multiple burns.

9. The patient is a five-year-old girl whose clothes caught fire while she was helping her mother bake cookies at home. She suffered first- and second-degree burns of her abdomen and right forearm. The physician dressed the burns and prescribed antibiotics. Impression: Burns of her abdomen and right forearm. How would this be coded?

T21.12XA	Burn of first degree of abdominal wall, initial encounter
T21.22XA	Burn of second degree of abdominal wall, initial encounter
T22.111A	Burn of first degree of right forearm, initial encounter
T22.211A	Burn of second degree of right forearm, initial encounter
T22.10XA	Burn of first degree of shoulder and upper limb, except wrist and hand, unspecified site, initial encounter
T22.20XA	Burn of second degree of shoulder and upper limb, except wrist and hand, unspecified site, initial encounter

   a. T21.22XA, T22.211A

   b. T21.12XA, T22.111A, T22.211A, T21.22XA

   c. T21.22XA, T22.20XA

   d. T21.12XA, T22.211A, T22.10XA

10. The patient is seen in the wound clinic for treatment of decubitus ulcers. The physician documents the final diagnoses as: Ulcer of left heel, stage 1; ulcer of right heel, stage 2. Which of the following codes would be reported?

   a. L89.621, L89.612

   b. L89.621

   c. L97.421, L97.412

   d. L89.622, L89.611

11. The 93-year-old female patient is admitted with confusion, tachycardia, fever, and tachypnea. The blood cultures were negative, but the physician documents the following final diagnoses: severe sepsis, septic shock, and respiratory failure. Which of the following codes would be reported?

   a. A41.9, R65.21, J96.00, R41.0, R50.9, R00.0, R06.82

   b. A41.89, R65.21, J96.00

   c. R65.21, J96.00

   d. A41.9, R65.21, J96.00

12. The coding guideline for coding sequelae is:

   a. Only the residual condition or nature of the sequela is coded

   b. The cause of the sequela is sequenced first followed by the residual condition

   c. Only the cause of the sequela is coded

   d. The residual condition is sequenced first, followed by the cause of the sequela

13. Full-thickness skin loss involving damage or necrosis into subcutaneous soft tissues describes which stage of decubitus ulcer?

   a. Stage I

   b. Stage II

   c. Stage III

   d. Stage IV

14. During a previous admission, the patient was diagnosed with adenocarcinoma of the body of the pancreas. She is being seen now for her third radiotherapy treatment. Which of the following codes would be reported?

    a. Z51.0, C25.1

    b. Z51.0

    c. C25.1

    d. C25.1, Z51.0

15. If a patient with a documented history of HIV disease is managed with antiretroviral medications, which coding selection meets the guidelines for coding?

    a. B20, Z79.899

    b. Z21, Z79.899

    c. R75, Z79.899

    d. B97.35

16. Which of the following is true about coding a COVID-19 infection?

    a. Confirmation of the COVID-19 infection requires documentation of a positive test result.

    b. If the provider documents probable or possible COVID-19, assign code U07.1, COVID-19.

    c. If the reason for an encounter is a complication or manifestation of COVID-19, the manifestation should be coded first.

    d. Code only a confirmed diagnosis of the 2019 novel coronavirus disease (COVID-19).

Domain 2 *Procedure Coding*

17. The patient reports pain, swelling, and the feeling of warmth in the ankle. The physician aspirates 12 cc of fluid from a cyst in the patient's ankle joint. How is this procedure coded?

    a. 10021, Fine needle aspiration biopsy, without imaging guidance; first lesion; without imaging guidance

    b. 20605, Arthrocentesis, aspiration and/or injection, intermediate joint of bursa (eg, temporomandibular, acromioclavicular, wrist, elbow or ankle, olecranon bursa); without ultrasound guidance

    c. 20615, Aspiration and injection for treatment of bone cyst

    d. 27604, Incision and drainage, leg or ankle; infected bursa

18. A portion of a patient's kidney is removed using an incisional technique. How is this service coded?

    a. 50045, Nephrotomy, with exploration

    b. 50240, Nephrectomy, partial

    c. 50340, Recipient nephrectomy (separate procedure)

    d. 50543, Laparoscopy, surgical; partial nephrectomy

19. The patient has a misaligned phalangeal shaft fracture demonstrated on a two-view x-ray, performed and read by the physician in the office. The physician manipulates the finger into alignment and places a rigid finger splint. How are these services coded?

26720	Closed treatment of phalangeal shaft fracture, proximal or middle phalanx, finger or thumb; without manipulation, each
26725	with manipulation, with or without skin or skeletal traction, each
26727	Percutaneous skeletal fixation of unstable phalangeal shaft fracture, proximal or middle phalanx, finger or thumb, with manipulation, each
73120	Radiologic examination, hand; 2 views
73140	Radiologic examination, finger(s), minimum of 2 views

    a. 26720, 73120

    b. 26725, 73120

    c. 26725, 73140

    d. 26727, 73140

20. The patient undergoes a revision tympanoplasty without ossicular chain reconstruction and a mastoidectomy. How is this service coded?

    a. 69631

    b. 69631, 69502

    c. 69635

    d. 69641

21. A 36-year-old male patient is taken to the operating room, and a central venous catheter is tunneled through the subclavian vein and terminated in the superior vena cava. How is this catheter insertion coded?

    a. 36557

    b. 36558

    c. 36569

    d. 36571

22. The patient has a blocked right iliac artery that cannot be opened. Therefore, the patient undergoes a left femoral artery bypass to the right femoral artery with a Gore-Tex prosthetic graft. The right femoral artery still does not show adequate back bleeding. A thromboendarterectomy is performed on the right common femoral artery. Adequate blood flow is achieved, and the anastomosis is completed. What is the correct coding for this procedure?

34201	Embolectomy or thrombectomy, without or without catheter; femoropopliteal, aortoiliac artery, by leg incision
35371	Thromboendarterectomy, including patch graft, if performed; common femoral
35558	Bypass graft, with vein; femoral-femoral
35621	Bypass graft, with other than vein; axillary-femoral
35661	Bypass graft, with other than vein; femoral-femoral

    a. 34201, 35558

    b. 34201, 35621

    c. 35371, 35558

    d. 35371, 35661

23. Which of the following codes is assigned to report electronic analysis, reprogramming, and refill of implanted intrathecal pump, performed by a pump technician under the general supervision of a physician?

    a. 62369, Electronic analysis of programmable, implanted pump for intrathecal or epidural drug infusion (includes evaluation of reservoir status, alarm status, drug prescription status); with reprogramming and refill

    b. 62370, Electronic analysis of programmable, implanted pump for intrathecal or epidural drug infusion (includes evaluation of reservoir status, alarm status, drug prescription status); with reprogramming and refill (requiring skill of a physician or other qualified health care professional)

    c. 95990, Refilling and maintenance of implantable pump or reservoir for drug delivery, spinal (intrathecal, epidural) or brain (intraventricular), includes electronic analysis of pump, when performed

    d. 95991, Refilling and maintenance of implantable pump or reservoir for drug delivery, spinal (intrathecal, epidural) or brain (intraventricular), includes electronic analysis of pump, when performed; requiring skill of a physician or other qualified health care professional

24. The patient is diagnosed with a fracture. The surgeon performed an open reduction of the right tibial fracture of the medial and posterior malleoli and used internal fixation. The surgeon also identified a syndesmosis disruption of the right ankle and performed an open repair with internal fixation. How is this coded?

    a. 27766, 27769, 27829
    b. 27810, 27818
    c. 27814, 27829
    d. 27848

25. The surgeon performs a percutaneous transcatheter mitral valve insertion (TMVI) using a transseptal puncture. How is this coded?

    a. 0483T
    b. 0484T
    c. 33418
    d. 33430

26. The patient (not covered by Medicare) is sent to a dermatologist by her primary care physician for diagnosis of a suspicious rash. A detailed history and examination are done, a biopsy is taken, and medication is prescribed. Medical decision-making is of low complexity. The physician spends 32 total minutes with the patient. The findings are sent back to the primary care physician. How is this E/M service coded?

    a. 99203
    b. 99214
    c. 99243
    d. 99254

27. A new patient is seen for a cough. The physician completes a detailed history and exam and documents low-level medical decision-making in evaluating the patient. An albuterol 2.5 mg and Atrovent 0.5 mg nebulizer treatment was given, and MDI teaching was performed. What is the correct code assignment for this case?

    a. 99202, 94640, J7611, J7644
    b. 99203, 94640, J7611, J7644
    c. 99204, 94640, 94664, J7620
    d. 99203, 94640, 94664, J7620

28. Patient undergoes percutaneous transluminal coronary balloon angioplasty of the right coronary artery, followed by stent placement at the site of the blockage. What is the correct code assignment?

    a. 92928-RC

    b. 92928-RC, 92920-RC

    c. 92928-RC, 92921-RC

    d. 92920-RC, 92928-RC

29. A patient's family practitioner referred him to a urologist for urinary incontinence. The problem was resolved, and the patient returned to his family practice physician. Two years later, the patient presents to the same urologist's office for problems with erectile dysfunction. The urologist performs a comprehensive history and exam. He documents 45 minutes spent with the patient. How would this case be coded?

    a. 99204

    b. 99214

    c. 99215

    d. 99244

30. A non-Medicare patient is referred by her regular physician to an ENT. She presents to the consultant's office with complaints of a cold. She has had a worsening stuffy nose and a sore throat since last week. She denies any cough, chest pain, or difficulty breathing. She has had an intermittent fever and admits feeling generally fatigued. She has no chronic health conditions. What level of history would be assigned to this case?

    a. Problem-focused

    b. Expanded problem-focused

    c. Detailed

    d. Comprehensive

31. When the physician's office performs a bilateral hand x-ray and the physician interprets the x-ray, what modifier(s) are required on the claim?

Modifier	Description
-26	Professional component
-50	Bilateral procedure
-51	Multiple procedure
-LT	Left side
-RT	Right side
-TC	Technical component

    a. -50

    b. -TC, -51

    c. -LT, -RT

    d. -26, -LT, -RT

32. The pathologist does a gross and microscopic examination on three surgical specimens from a bronchoscopy procedure. Specimens submitted were biopsies of lung, bronchus, and trachea. The pathologist is not employed by the hospital. What is the correct code assignment for the services of the pathologist?

> | 88300 | Level I—Surgical pathology, gross examination only |
> | 88305 | Level IV—Surgical pathology, gross and microscopic examination |
> | -26 | Professional component |
> | -TC | Technical component |

    a. 88300, 88305

    b. 88305-26

    c. 88305-26 ×3

    d. 88300-TC, 88300-TC, 88305-TC

33. The physician saw the patient in the hospital and a flexible bronchoscopy with therapeutic aspiration was performed in the trachea and both the left and right main bronchi today. This is the second flexible bronchoscopy performed to aspirate secretions from the lungs during this hospital admission. How is this coded?

    a. 31622

    b. 31624-76

    c. 31645-76

    d. 31646

34. Which of the following is required for the billing of Transitional Care Management (TCM) Services?

    a. A face-to-face visit with at least moderate medical decision-making takes place within two business days of the hospital discharge.

    b. An interactive contact takes place with the patient within two business days of the hospital discharge.

    c. The patient is admitted to a skilled nursing facility directly from the hospital.

    d. The patient is discharged from a skilled nursing facility to his or her own home, domiciliary, rest home, or assisted living facility.

35. The patient presented for wound debridement. The physician debrided a 10 sq cm wound on the patient's left thigh that extended into the muscle. Next, the physician debrided a 5 sq cm wound on the left calf, which also extended into the muscle. A third wound, measuring 9 sq cm and extending into the muscle of the left arm, was then debrided. Lastly, a 8 sq cm wound extending into the bone of the left shoulder was debrided. How would this be coded?

    a. 11043, 11044

    b. 11044, 11043

    c. 11043, 11043, 11043, 11044

    d. 11044, 11043, 11046

36. A patient presents for a diagnostic nasal sinus endoscopy. During the course of the procedure, the physician performs a sinusotomy and total ethmoidectomy. How is this procedure coded?

    a. 31231, 31020

    b. 31255, 31231, 31020

    c. 31255, 31020

    d. 31255

37. A patient presents to her oncologist's office for IV infusion of chemotherapy, which is administered to the patient over one hour. The physician feels that the patient could also benefit from IV hydration, which is then administered over 45 minutes. In addition to the HCPCS Level II code for the drug, how would this service be coded?

    a. 96360, 96413

    b. 96360, 96415

    c. 96413, 96360

    d. 96413, 96361

38. What is the proper code assignment when the documentation states simple wound repair of three arm lacerations at 1.5 cm, 3.0 cm, and 4.0 cm and intermediate wound repair of two hand lacerations at 1.5 cm and 2.0 cm?

12001	Simple repair of superficial wounds of scalp, neck, axillae, external genitalia, trunk and/or extremities (including hands and feet); 2.5 cm or less
12002	2.6 cm to 7.5 cm
12004	7.6 cm to 12.5 cm
12005	12.6 cm to 20.0 cm
12041	Repair, intermediate, wounds of neck, hands, feet and/or external genitalia; 2.5 cm or less
12042	2.6 cm to 7.5 cm
12044	7.6 cm to 12.5 cm

    a. 12042, 12004

    b. 12044

    c. 12005

    d. 12041, 12041, 12001, 12002, 12002

39. The physician excises two benign lesions measuring 0.5 cm and 2.0 cm from the patient's shoulder. Each excision site was closed with a simple repair. How should the coding professional code this service?

    a. Code the excision of a 2.5 cm lesion.

    b. Code the excision of a 2.5 cm lesion and a 2.5 cm simple repair.

    c. Code the excision of a 0.5 cm lesion and a 2.0 cm lesion.

    d. Code the excision of each lesion separately and the simple repairs separately.

40. An internal medicine physician requests an orthopedic physician to see his patient, who is not covered by Medicare. The patient fell out of the bed trying to go the restroom. The patient is unable to bear weight on her left foot. The orthopedic physician examines the patient, orders and review x-rays, and reports his findings to the internal medicine physician. The patient is taken to surgery later in the day for a hip reduction. How is the initial orthopedic visit coded?

    a. It is coded as an inpatient consultation with modifier 57 (Decision for Surgery).

    b. It is coded as an initial hospital visit with modifier 57.

    c. It is coded as an initial hospital visit without modifier 57.

    d. It is not coded at all; the orthopedic surgeon bills for the surgery.

41. A patient undergoes a thoracotomy with a diagnostic biopsy of lung nodules. Upon further examination during the same operative episode, the physician elects to proceed with a lobectomy. How would this be coded?

    a. Code the biopsy only.

    b. Code the lobectomy only.

    c. Code the biopsy and the lobectomy with modifier 51.

    d. Code the biopsy and the lobectomy with modifier 58.

42. According to the National Correct Coding Initiative (NCCI), how should a bilateral procedure code be reported?

    a. Report the code only once with modifier 50.

    b. Report the code twice.

    c. Report the code with two units of service.

    d. Report the code twice with modifiers LT and RT.

43. A patient presents to her regular physician's office with complaints of post-menopausal bleeding and a family history of uterine cancer. The physician documents a medically appropriate history and physical. He schedules the patient for a hysteroscopy and D&C. Based on the diagnoses and plan, what E/M code should be reported?

99203	Office or other outpatient visit for the evaluation and management of a new patient, which requires a medically appropriate history and/or examination and low level of medical decision making
99204	Office or other outpatient visit for the evaluation and management of a new patient, which requires a medically appropriate history and/or examination and moderate level of medical decision making
99213	Office or other outpatient visit for the evaluation and management of an established patient, which requires a medically appropriate history and/or examination and low level of medical decision making
99214	Office or other outpatient visit for the evaluation and management of an established patient, which requires a medically appropriate history and/or examination and moderate level of medical decision making

    a. 99203

    b. 99204

    c. 99213

    d. 99214

44. The patient undergoes removal of a 2 cm lipoma of the soft tissue of the back. How would this be coded?

11302	Shaving of epidermal or dermal lesion, single lesion, trunk, arms, or legs; lesion diameter 1.1 to 2.0 cm
11402	Excision, benign lesion including margins, except skin tag (unless listed elsewhere), trunk, arms, or legs; excised diameter 1.1 to 2.0 cm
11602	Excision, malignant lesion including margins, trunk, arms, or legs; excised diameter 1.1 to 2.0 cm
21930	Excision, tumor, soft tissue of back or flank, subcutaneous; less than 3 cm

a. 11302

b. 11402

c. 11602

d. 21930

45. The statement of procedure in an operative note says: "Biopsy of suspected malignant lesion of left breast." The body of the operative report indicates incision with removal of the entire suspicious lesion. How would this procedure be classified?

a. Percutaneous breast biopsy

b. Excision of breast lesion

c. Percutaneous breast biopsy with localization device

d. Incisional breast biopsy

46. A patient receives a one hour infusion of Vancomycin. How would this be coded?

a. Assign a code for hydration, therapeutic infusion, and a drug code for the Vancomycin.

b. Assign a code for therapeutic infusion, and a drug code for the Vancomycin.

c. Assign a code for chemotherapy and other highly complex drug administration, and a drug code for the Vancomycin.

d. Assign the drug code for Vancomycin only.

47. The physician performs a colonoscopy on a 30-year-old male. He notes ulcers in the rectum and takes several biopsies. How would this be coded?

45100	Biopsy of anorectal wall, anal approach (eg, congenital megacolon)
45378	Colonoscopy, flexible; diagnostic, including collection of specimens by brushing or washing when performed (separate procedure)
45380	with biopsy, single or multiple
45384	with removal of tumor(s), polyp(s), or other lesion(s) by hot biopsy forceps

a. 45100

b. 45378, 45100

c. 45380

d. 45384

48. The physician performs a transanal hemorrhoidal dearterization (THD) using an anoscope with Doppler guidance to identify hemorrhoidal arteries supplying two columns of internal hemorrhoids, and ties them off with sutures. How would this be coded?

46615	Anoscopy; with ablation of tumor(s), polyp(s), or other lesion(s) not amenable to removal by hot biopsy forceps, bipolar cautery or snare technique
46930	Destruction of internal hemorrhoid(s) by thermal energy (eg, infrared coagulation, cautery, radiofrequency)
46946	Hemorrhoidectomy, internal, by ligation other than rubber band; 2 or more hemorrhoid columns/groups, without imaging guidance
46948	Hemorrhoidectomy, internal, by transanal hemorrhoidal dearterialization, 2 or more hemorrhoid columns/groups including ultrasound guidance, with mucopexy, when performed

  a. 46615

  b. 46930

  c. 46946

  d. 46948

Domain 3 *Research*

49. Which of the following is excluded from the surgical global?

  a. Consultation to determine the need for procedure

  b. Local, regional, or topical anesthesia administered

  c. The surgical procedure performed

  d. Routine postoperative follow-up care

50. A patient is seen in the physician's office with a diagnosis of hypertensive crisis. The physician has been treating the patient for hypertension for several years. The patient's current blood pressure is 210/100. The physician would report the following codes:

I10	Essential (primary) hypertension
I16.1	Hypertensive emergency
I16.9	Hypertensive crisis, unspecified
R03.0	Elevated blood-pressure reading, without diagnosis of hypertension

  a. I16.9

  b. I16.9; R03.0

  c. I16.1; I10

  d. I16.9; I10

51. A physician examines a patient for congestive heart failure. The patient is known to have a hiatal hernia and arthritis. The congestive heart failure is evaluated, blood pressure recorded, and medications adjusted for the congestive heart failure and the hypertension. What conditions are reportable?

    a. Congestive heart failure

    b. Congestive heart failure; hypertension

    c. Congestive heart failure; hypertension; arthritis

    d. Congestive heart failure; hypertension; arthritis; hiatal hernia

52. A coding professional uses local coverage determinations (LCDs) from Medicare to identify:

    a. Which procedures require prior approval before payment is made by the third party

    b. Which ICD-10-CM codes justify the medical necessity of a test or service

    c. The reimbursement for a specific procedure

    d. Which ICD-10-PCS codes justify the medical necessity of a test or service

53. Many evaluation and management code descriptions mention various levels of history, examination, and medical decision-making. What official source can coding professionals use to determine which level is described by the documentation in the health record?

    a. Physician queries

    b. National Correct Coding Initiative

    c. AHIMA textbooks

    d. Documentation Guidelines

54. A coding professional is assigning a code for an IM injection of a therapeutic medication. She finds the code for the injection itself in the CPT manual but is unsure how to proceed from there. The coding professional should:

    a. Stop there—coding for the encounter is complete.

    b. Seek an unlisted procedure code in the Medicine section to report along with the code for the injection.

    c. Seek a general supplies and equipment code in the CPT manual.

    d. Consult the HCPCS Level II national codes to determine a specific code for the drug administered.

55. Dr. Smith provides all of the antenatal care to his patient Mary Dinu prior to her moving to another state. Her new physician, Dr. Jones, delivers her baby and the placental products vaginally, and provides all postpartum care. What is the proper coding for Dr. Jones?

    a. 59400-52

    b. 59409, 59430

    c. 59410, 59414

    d. 59410

56. Which of the following is an example of a leading query?

    a. The consulting pulmonologist documents pneumonia as an impression based on the chest x-ray. Do you agree with the pulmonologist's diagnosis of pneumonia?

    b. Please review the laboratory section of the health record to confirm your discharge diagnosis of hypernatremia. Laboratory findings indicate a serum sodium of 120 mmol/L.

    c. Is the patient's pneumonia due to aspiration? This seems to be indicated by clinical findings.

    d. Please clarify your diagnosis of "no intraoperative complications." The operative note indicates "cautery lesion to lip."

57. Review the following physician query:

    DOCUMENTATION CLARIFICATION REQUEST

    Patient Name: Grey Emerson

    Please document in your next progress note or discharge summary or click on "REPLY" and type your response to this query.
    On 1-1-20XX, pneumonia was documented in the medical record in the progress notes.

    Clinical Indicators:
    - Physical symptoms (fever, cough, SOB, RR, HR, O_2 needs)
    - Lab values (WBC, bands, procalcitonin, hsCRP, Sputum Cx)
    - Radiology (CXR, CT chest)
    - Swallow study results
    - Treatment (antibiotics, resp therapy, bipap, vent, O_2)
    - Other

    Based on your medical judgment, please indicate if any of the following diagnoses are appropriate for this patient.
    - ☐ Aspiration pneumonia
    - ☐ Bacterial pneumonia (please specify known or suspected organism)
    - ☐ Community-acquired pneumonia
    - ☐ Gram negative pneumonia (specify known or suspected organism)
    - ☐ Gram positive pneumonia (specify known or suspected organism)
    - ☐ Healthcare-associated pneumonia
    - ☐ Viral pneumonia
    - ☐ No pneumonia present
    - ☐ Other _____
    - ☐ Unable to determine

    Which is *not* true about the physician query form?

    a. It is sent to determine more specific information about the pneumonia.

    b. It would be considered a leading query.

    c. It would be considered a nonleading query.

    d. Multiple choice format is appropriate for a physician query.

58. Given the following information, which of the statements is most appropriate to use in the physician query?

    Clinical Indicators: A patient is admitted for a right hip fracture. The H&P notes that the patient has a history of chronic congestive heart failure. The echocardiogram showed an ejection fraction (left ventricular) of 25 percent. The patient's home medications include metoprolol and Lasix.

    a. Please document if you agree that the patient has chronic diastolic heart failure.

    b. It is noted in the H&P that the patient has congestive heart failure. Can you further specify the type of chronic heart failure?

    c. Would you add a diagnosis of diastolic heart failure to your discharge summary?

    d. Does the documentation support a diagnosis of chronic systolic heart failure?

59. Where would a coding professional who needed to locate the histology of a documented breast cancer most likely find this information?

    a. Pathology report

    b. Progress notes

    c. Nurse's notes

    d. Operative report

60. Where would information on treatment given during a specific encounter be found in the health record?

    a. Problem list

    b. Physician's orders

    c. Progress notes

    d. Physical examination

61. A patient is admitted with acute cholecystitis. The physician notes in the History and Physical that the patient has a history of pneumonia two years ago and status post bunionectomy earlier that year. The physician documents on the discharge summary: acute cholecystitis, history of pneumonia, and bunionectomy. How should the admission be reported?

    a. Acute cholecystitis

    b. Acute cholecystitis and pneumonia

    c. Cholecystitis and status post bunionectomy

    d. Acute cholecystitis, pneumonia, and status post bunionectomy

62. The coding professional notes that on the patient's laboratory results, the hemoglobin is 7.3 g/dL. The physician orders iron supplements. What should the coding professional report?

    a. Abnormal laboratory findings

    b. Iron-deficiency anemia

    c. Hemorrhaging

    d. The coding professional should query the physician to ask him to add an appropriate diagnosis

63. This federal agency develops an annual healthcare work plan:

    a. IRS

    b. FBI

    c. DEA

    d. OIG

64. A program unveiled by the Office of the Inspector General that expanded and simplified methods for healthcare providers to voluntarily report fraudulent conduct affecting Medicare, Medicaid, and other federal healthcare programs is the:

    a. Provider Self-Disclosure Protocol

    b. Federal False Claims Act

    c. Operation Restore Trust

    d. Health Insurance Portability and Accountability Act

65. HIM staff notices that the physician failed to sign all of the patient's progress notes prior to discharge. Upon discharge, the record is considered:

    a. Closed

    b. Open

    c. Incomplete

    d. Delinquent

66. The diagnosis of "allergic reaction to unknown drug taken as prescribed" would be a(n):

    a. Adverse effect

    b. Late effect

    c. Poisoning

    d. Misadventure

67. The patient was admitted to the hospital for moderate-stage primary low tension open angle glaucoma of the right and left eyes. The right eye was controlled, but the left eye progressed to severe-stage glaucoma. What is the correct diagnosis code for the physician's services?

H40.121	Low-tension, glaucoma, right eye
H40.122	Low-tension, glaucoma, left eye
H40.123	Low-tension, glaucoma, bilateral
	0 stage unspecified
	1 mild stage
	2 moderate stage
	3 severe stage
	4 indeterminate stage

    a. H40.1212, H40.1222

    b. H40.1212, H40.1223

    c. H40.1232

    d. H40.1233

68. The patient is seen by his nephrologist for stage 1 CKD. The patient had a kidney transplant six years ago. Which diagnosis codes are submitted for this encounter?

> N18.1   Chronic kidney disease, stage 1
> T86.10   Unspecified complication of kidney transplant
> Z94.0   Kidney transplant status
> Z90.5   Acquired absence of kidney

    a. N18.1, Z94.0, Z90.5

    b. N18.1, T86.10, Z94.0

    c. N18.1, Z94.0

    d. N18.1, T86.10

69. Within the CMS-HCC model, individual HCCs are valid for how many years?

    a. No limit on number of years

    b. One year

    c. Two years

    d. Three years

70. HCC models use several primary sources of data to determine a person's risk adjustment factor (RAF). Which of the following is not a data source used in determining the patient's RAF?

    a. Patient's age

    b. Patient's gender

    c. ICD-10-CM diagnosis codes

    d. ICD-10-PCS procedure codes

71. The Minimum Necessary Rule refers to which of the following?

    a. Copying all billing and medical records as requested by the patient

    b. Releasing copies of the entire medical record for all disclosure requests

    c. Disclosing personal health information is held to the smallest amount of information necessary to accomplish the intended purpose of the use or disclosure

    d. Requesting personal health information by public officials who have a right to the information as dictated by state law

72. Although the HIPAA Privacy Rule allows patients access to personal health information about themselves, which of the following *cannot* be disclosed to patients?

    a. Interpretation of x-rays by the radiologist

    b. Billing records

    c. Progress notes written by the attending physician

    d. Psychotherapy notes

73. The HIPAA Security Rule applies to:

    a. All PHI

    b. ePHI

    c. Deidentified health information

    d. Aggregate health information

74. According to the Security Rule, security awareness training is considered what type of safeguard?

    a. Administrative

    b. Technical

    c. Physical

    d. Policy

75. A patient is admitted with respiratory failure and shortness of breath following a previous admission for COVID-19. The patient tests negative for COVID-19. The physician documents "Pulmonary embolism due to previous COVID-19 infection." What diagnosis codes are reported for this admission?

    a. I26.99, U07.1

    b. I26.99, U09.9

    c. I26.99, B94.8, Z20.828

    d. I26.99, B94.8, U07.1

76. The 86-year-old patient is seen by the physician one month posthospitalization for COVID-19 as a precautionary measure. Her current COVID-19 test is negative. Her glucose levels were normal; she is a type 2 diabetic with neuralgia who has been on insulin for many years. What diagnosis codes should be reported for this encounter?

    a. Z86.19, E11.42, Z79.4

    b. Z09, Z86.19, E11.42

    c. Z09, Z86.19, E11.9, Z79.4

    d. Z09, Z86.19, E11.42, Z79.4

77. In relation to Practice Expense in the Resource-based Relative Value Scale (RBRVS), which of the following is considered a facility?

    a. Ambulatory surgical center

    b. Physician's office

    c. Urgent care center

    d. Dialysis center

78. Which of the following should be considered in determining the place of service for procedure?

    a. Patient's medical condition

    b. Type of procedure

    c. Patient's preference

    d. All of the above

79. Initial Visit: A physician sees Ms. Richard for high blood pressure. She prescribes medication and a 1,500-calorie diet as part of a long-term treatment plan; Ms. Richard is to have her blood pressure checked in the office every four weeks. On the second visit, Ms. Richard has her blood pressure checked by the Advanced Practice Registered Nurse (APRN) because the physician is on vacation. How would this office visit be billed?

    a. The claim would be submitted using the physician's National Provider Identifier (NPI).

    b. No claim would be submitted just for a blood pressure check.

    c. The claim would be submitted using the APRN's NPI.

    d. A single claim would be submitted once every six months.

80. Initial Visit: A physician sees Ms. Richard for high blood pressure. She prescribes medication and a 1,500-calorie diet as part of a long-term treatment plan; Ms. Richard is to have her blood pressure checked in the office every four weeks. On the second visit, Ms Richard has her blood pressure checked by the Advanced Practice Registered Nurse (APRN) because the physician is on vacation. On the third visit, the physician is in the office but seeing another patient. The APRN checks her blood pressure. How would this third office visit be billed?

    a. The claim would be submitted using the physician's National Provider Identifier (NPI).

    b. No claim would be submitted just for a blood pressure check.

    c. The claim would be submitted using the APRN's NPI.

    d. A single claim would be submitted once every six months.

81. Which of the following Medicare integrity programs measures the numbers of improper payments in various provider settings?

    a. Recovery Audit Program (RAC)

    b. MAC quality reviews

    c. Comprehensive Error Rate Testing (CERT) program

    d. Value-based purchasing program

82. You are the coding supervisor at Acadia West Hospital and contracted with Medical Auditors to perform an outpatient claim audit for the clinics associated with the hospital. The final report showed that the coding professionals were billing for more complex services than those that were actually documented in the health record. What type of coding error did Medical Auditors discover?

    a. Unbundling

    b. Upcoding

    c. Optimizing

    d. Exploding

83. Which type of compliance documents is used by Medicare to communicate the circumstances under which supplies, services, or procedures are covered nationwide by Medicare?

    a. CMS program transmittals

    b. National coverage determinations

    c. Local coverage determinations

    d. National Correct Coding Initiative

84. The compliance analyst at your facility is preparing an audit plan for the upcoming quarter. She has decided that she will select health records to audit by reviewing the health record numbers for admissions during the quarter. She will select the first number on the list and every fifth one after that. Which probability sampling technique will the analyst be using for this audit?

    a. Simple random sampling

    b. Cluster sampling

    c. Stratified random sampling

    d. Systematic random sampling

85. The compliance analyst at your physician practice facility is preparing an audit plan for the upcoming quarter. She is concerned that the coding professionals are not selecting the appropriate first-listed diagnosis in all cases. The quality rate she has selected will include the correct first-listed diagnosis code having a higher weight than other codes. Which type of compliance rate methodology is the analyst planning to use?

    a. Code over code

    b. Weighted code over code

    c. Record over record

    d. Weighted record over record

86. As the denial specialist at your practice, you are reviewing a denial where the third-party payer denial was based on insufficient clinical indicators documented to support a diagnosis of sepsis. What type of denial is this?

    a. Administrative

    b. Clinical

    c. Clinical validation

    d. Administrative validation

Domain 5 *Revenue Cycle*

87. Which of the following is *not* a main purpose of clinical documentation?

    a. Improved patient care through clear communication

    b. Accurate picture of patient's medical situation and course of treatment

    c. Accounting of disclosures for HIPAA requirements

    d. Review of patient safety measures

88. What is a claim called that contains all required data elements needed to process and pay the claim quickly?

    a. Open

    b. Clean

    c. Closed

    d. Final

89. When payments are made to the provider by EFT, this means that the reimbursement is:

    a. Sent to the provider's bank electronically

    b. Sent to the patient who will pay the provider

    c. Sent to the provider by check

    d. Sent to the managed care company electronically

90. Which of the following documents would not be used to reconcile payment for services provided to a patient?

    a. Explanation of benefits

    b. Remittance advice

    c. Medicare Summary Notice

    d. Outpatient Code Editor

91. The amount that a nonparticipating (nonPAR) physician who does not accept assignment can bill a Medicare beneficiary is called the:

    a. NonPAR value

    b. Contractual limit

    c. Limiting charge

    d. Nonassigned charge

92. The patient is seen at Wolf Place Physician Practice. The total charge for the visit is $250.00. The physician is a participating (PAR) physician and the patient has met the deductible for 20XX. The Medicare fee schedule amount for the E/M code is $200.00. What is the amount that the federal government will reimburse the physician?

    a. $250.00

    b. $200.00

    c. $190.00

    d. $160.00

93. What diagnoses and procedures should be reported for recurrent left inguinal hernia with laparoscopic repair?

    a. K40.91, 49520

    b. K40.31, 49521

    c. K40.91, 49651

    d. K40.30, 49520

94. The following coding was reviewed by the coding manager before the claims were submitted. What change would the coding manager request to help ensure payment?

Case	CPT Code(s)	Description	Diagnosis	Description
1	90713 90471	Poliovirus vaccine, inactivated (IPV), for subcutaneous or intramuscular use Immunization administration; 1 vaccine	Z23	Encounter for immunization
2	82465 73030	Cholesterol serum or whole blood, total Radiologic examination, shoulder; complete, minimum of 2 views	M25.512 E78.00	Pain in left shoulder Pure hypercholesterolemia, unspecified

a. Modifiers should be placed on the CPT codes.

b. Code the diagnoses codes to a greater level of specificity.

c. Additional CPT codes are required to describe the service.

d. Link the diagnoses codes correctly to the procedures.

95. Dr. Emerson's claim for patient John Doe, age 55, was denied by the insurance company. The final diagnosis code was I05.9, Rheumatic mitral valve disease, unspecified, and the service performed was 33206, Insertion of new or replacement of permanent pacemaker with transvenous electrode(s); atrial. This was a replacement of a pacemaker that was inserted two years ago. The most probably cause of the denial is:

a. Pacemaker placement is prohibited with the patient's age

b. Medical necessity was not shown by the diagnosis

c. An additional CPT code should be used to show the insertion of the lead into the atria

d. There must a five-year time period between pacemaker insertions or replacements

96. A measure that assesses the ability to comply with documentation, coding, and billing requirements is the:

a. Denial rate

b. Clean claim rate

c. PEPPER rate

d. Capture rate

97. For which group of clinicians is the RBRVS modified by base units and time?

a. General practitioners

b. Surgeons

c. Anesthesiologists

d. Nurse practitioners

Multiple Choice Exam 3 Answers

1.	26.	51.	76.
2.	27.	52.	77.
3.	28.	53.	78.
4.	29.	54.	79.
5.	30.	55.	80.
6.	31.	56.	81.
7.	32.	57.	82.
8.	33.	58.	83.
9.	34.	59.	84.
10.	35.	60.	85.
11.	36.	61.	86.
12.	37.	62.	87.
13.	38.	63.	88.
14.	39.	64.	89.
15.	40.	65.	90.
16.	41.	66.	91.
17.	42.	67.	92.
18.	43.	68.	93.
19.	44.	69.	94.
20.	45.	70.	95.
21.	46.	71.	96.
22.	47.	72.	97.
23.	48.	73.	
24.	49.	74.	
25.	50.	75.	

EXAM 3 MEDICAL SCENARIOS

EXAM 3—SCENARIO 1

REQUESTING PHYSICIAN: Dr. Z, Primary Care

HISTORY: This is a very pleasant 63-year-old white male with multiple past medical histories who is seen initially with the chief complaint of altered mental status at the nursing home. An infectious disease consult has been obtained for a possible urinary tract infection and sepsis.

SOCIAL HISTORY: The patient is a nursing home resident here.

MEDICATIONS: Avonex and Norvasc

ALLERGIES: None

REVIEW OF SYSTEMS: Pertinent for altered mental status

PHYSICAL EXAMINATION:

VITAL SIGNS: The patient is currently afebrile. Blood pressure 152/94.

GENERAL: The patient is in no distress. Alert, awake, and oriented times two.

CARDIOVASCULAR: Regular rate and rhythm. Positive S1 and S2. No murmurs.

LUNGS: Clear to auscultation. No wheezes or crackles.

ABDOMEN: Bowel sounds positive. Nontender.

EXTREMITIES: Good pulses. No edema.

LABORATORY DATA: Urinalysis positive for pyuria. Urine culture with gram-negative, anaerobic *Providencia stuartii*.

ASSESSMENT:

1. Sepsis due to *Providencia stuartii*

2. Urinary tract infection

RECOMMENDATIONS:

1. Recommend starting the patient on Rocephin.

2. Check blood cultures times two sets.

Thank you for recommending this consultation. Please fax a copy to Dr. Z's office.

HISTORY: Detailed

EXAMINATION: Detailed

MEDICAL DECISION-MAKING: Moderate

Enter three diagnosis codes and one procedure code.

DX1

DX2

DX3

PR1

EXAM 3—SCENARIO 2

SERVICE: Trauma service

HPI: This patient arrived at the emergency department on 10/07/20XX at approximately 19:00. The patient is a 25-year-old Hispanic female who is status post pedestrian versus motor vehicle collision. The patient reports a questionable loss of consciousness prior to arrival. Upon arrival the patient's prehospital blood pressure was noted to be 130/90 with prehospital heart rate of 126. The patient was in severe pain, complaining of pain mostly over the left anterior chest wall and of the left leg, and was admitted to trauma service. Upon questioning the patient denied allergies.

PAST MEDICAL HISTORY: Normal

MEDICATIONS: None

PAST SURGICAL HISTORY: Significant for removal of the gallbladder

FAMILY HISTORY: Normal

SOCIAL HISTORY: Occasional use of alcohol, approximately 2 to 3 drinks per week, but the patient denied use of tobacco or illicit drugs.

REVIEW OF SYSTEMS: No fever or fatigue; no systemic complaints. The patient's dermatologic review of systems was negative. She reports no rashes or any outstanding skin conditions. The patient's ear, nose, and throat review of systems was also unremarkable. The patient's cardiovascular, pulmonary, and gastrointestinal systems were all unremarkable with no specific complaints toward chest pain, shortness of breath, or change in bowel habits. Additionally, the patient's musculoskeletal review of systems was normal without prior history of musculoskeletal disease or weakness. The patient's genitourinary review of systems was normal with no complaints of dysuria, abnormal genitalia, burning, or itching. Psychiatric and neurologic review of systems was also unremarkable. The patient's skin was unremarkable historically but upon presentation the patient did complain of a rash and abrasion secondary to her trauma.

PRIMARY SURVEY: Clear airway that required no intervention. The patient arrived in C spine immobilization in a hard collar and backboard. The patient was found to be breathing spontaneously and unlabored.

Skin was warm, normal in color, without signs of external hemorrhage. The patient's carotid, femoral, radial, and dorsalis pedis pulses were all palpable and 2+ positive.

The patient was found to be alert, GCS approximately 14 with the only abnormality of the eyes not opening spontaneously and only to voice. Pupils were found to be reactive, 4-2, and symmetric. The patient's Glasgow coma scale upon initial evaluation in the trauma bay was that of GCS 14 and the patient's total trauma score was 12. The patient had a CT scan of the head, chest, abdomen, and pelvis, as well as reconstructed views of the cervical, thoracic, and lumbar spines performed. These scans were reviewed with the physician in the radiology department. The CT of the head was negative, with no obvious skull deformity or fracture, and no intracranial bleeding. Her chest revealed several abnormalities including a pulmonary contusion of the left upper lobe, hemopneumothorax, and depressed rib fractures at left ribs 2, 3, 4, 5, and 6. The rib fractures at 4 and 5 were comminuted. Rib 6 was severely displaced and crushed inward. However, upon evaluation of the CT scan there was no evidence or indication of thoracic vascular injury. CT scan of the abdomen was unremarkable. The patient's CT scan of the pelvis revealed left pubic rami fracture. The patient's cervical, thoracic, and lumbar spine images were reconstructed using the CT scan. These images revealed C spine, T spine, and L spine that were essentially without abnormality. The patient's point of care laboratory results included a hemoglobin of 14.1, sodium 143, potassium 3.6, chlorine 102, BUN 12, base excess of 2, pH 7.38, PO_2 37, PCO_2 45, lactate 1.9.

SECONDARY SURVEY: HEENT: The patient's pupils were equally round and reactive to light bilaterally, going from 4 mm to 2 mm with direct light stimulation. The patient's gaze was normal with tympanic

EXAM 3—SCENARIO 2 (*continued*)

membranes on the right and left clear. The oropharynx was found to be clear but tender at the chin. Gag reflex was intact and inclusion was normal. Neck revealed collapsed veins with trachea midline. There was no tenderness or crepitance in the neck. The chest revealed some external bilateral upper chest abrasions. The chest wall was seen to be symmetric; however, breath sounds were found to be abnormal with decreased breath sounds, particularly in the left chest. Heart sounds were regular rate and rhythm without murmurs, rubs, or gallops. The patient was not found to have crepitance of the chest wall. However, there was severe tenderness to palpation at the left anterior chest wall. Abdomen revealed no external trauma to the abdomen, no tenderness to palpation, obese yet normal contour to the abdomen. Abdomen was dull to percussion. Pelvis stable and nontender by examination. Genitourinary revealed no blood at the meatus and the urine pregnancy test was negative. Rectal revealed normal sphincter tone with brown stool. Spine revealed a nontender cervical, thoracic, and lumbar spine. There was no evidence of step-off deformity at any of these levels. Neuro revealed motor strength 5+/5+ in both right and left upper and lower extremities. Additionally, sensory examination revealed no deficits. Vascular exam revealed 2+ radial pulses bilaterally. Additionally, femoral, posterior tibial, and dorsalis pulses were all 2+ bilaterally.

ASSESSMENT: 25-year-old female involved in a pedestrian versus motor vehicle trauma. The patient suffered multiple injuries. The patient suffered rib fractures from ribs 2 to 6 on the left side. Ribs 4 and 5 on the left side were found to have the comminuted fractures with resultant hemopneumothorax and pulmonary contusion.

Rib 6 was also a severely displaced rib fracture with displacement into the thoracic cavity. Reconstructed images of the cervical, thoracic, and lumbar spines were negative. C spine showed questionable transverse fracture at level T4.

PLAN:

1. Watch respiratory status due to pulmonary insult. The patient is to receive IPPV treatments in the TICU.

2. Orthopedic consultation for the suprapubic ramus fracture.

ADDENDUM

REVISION TO ADMISSION H&P DICTATION: The patient had no evidence of fracture abnormality on her C spine on reconstructed images. Repeat, there was no abnormality on C spine, which was negative. This was cleared radiographically.

HISTORY: Comprehensive

EXAMINATION: Comprehensive

MEDICAL DECISION-MAKING: High

Enter four diagnosis codes and one procedure code.

DX1

DX2

DX3

DX4

PR1

EXAM 3—SCENARIO 3

PREOPERATIVE DIAGNOSIS: Conn's syndrome with abnormal aldosterone secretion from the left adrenal gland

POSTOPERATIVE DIAGNOSIS: Conn's syndrome with abnormal aldosterone secretion from the left adrenal gland

OPERATION PERFORMED: Laparoscopic left adrenalectomy

ATTENDING SURGEON:

ANESTHESIA: General

ESTIMATED BLOOD LOSS: Less than 20 cc

FLUID REPLACEMENT: 1,000 cc lactated Ringer's solution

URINE OUTPUT: 175 cc

SPECIMENS: Left adrenal gland

INDICATIONS FOR PROCEDURE: This 46-year-old African-American female has hypertension and hypokalemia. Her medications include Norvasc and potassium supplement. Workup revealed hyperaldosteronism that, after adrenal vein sampling, appeared to localize specifically to the left adrenal gland with markedly elevated levels of aldosterone. After the risks and benefits of the procedure and possible complications were explained, the patient elected to undergo laparoscopic left adrenalectomy.

DESCRIPTION OF PROCEDURE: The patient was brought to the operative suite and positioned on the operating room table in the right lateral decubitus position with the left side up. She was adequately padded and taped in position. She was then prepared and draped in the usual sterile fashion. Initial access to the abdomen was obtained using a direct cut-down technique below the left ribs. Insertion of a blunt cannula was undertaken and the abdomen was insufflated under direct visualization. There appeared to be limited working space in the abdomen due to the patient's central obesity and a large amount of intra-abdominal fat. In addition, the patient had a very large fatty liver that was clear over to the left abdomen. Under direct visualization, we placed a more medial 5.0-mm trocar in the left hypochondrium and in addition, two 5.0-mm trocars in the left hypochondrium more lateral to our initial access site.

We proceeded to mobilize the left colon from the left sidewall using harmonic shears, and we adequately mobilized the colon out of the way. We then proceeded to roll the colon mesentery medially where we could identify Gerota's fascia.

We then followed Gerota's fascia superiorly and rolled the inferior pole of the spleen medially and superiorly, rolling the spleen off its left lateral attachments. This allowed us to identify the area of the adrenal gland. We then proceeded to open up Gerota's fascia gently using an L-hook cautery and identified the adrenal gland in place, which appeared to be somewhat long and flat in appearance.

After Gerota's fascia was completely opened to expose the adrenal gland in its entirety, meticulous dissection was carried out inferiorly and medially, where we identified a solitary left adrenal vein, which we triply clipped and divided. Further L-hook cautery was then used to dissect the gland from the underlying fat. This was done with excellent hemostasis. Additional small blood vessels were clipped and divided, and further dissection enabled identification of the left phrenic vein, which again was triply clipped and divided. We then further dissected the adrenal gland off its bed using L-hook cautery with excellent hemostasis. We then placed the gland into an impermeable entrapment sac and removed it through the initial access site, passing it off the field. Inspection of the adrenal bed revealed it to have good hemostasis. We irrigated with warm normal saline and aspirated back. There was no evidence of bleeding. We then proceeded to close our initial access trocar site with 0 Vicryl suture on a suture-passer using a figure-of-8 technique. The rest of the abdomen was inspected. We replaced the left colon back into the left upper abdomen. There was no injury to the colon throughout the entire procedure. The patient tolerated the procedure well.

EXAM 3—SCENARIO 3 (*continued*)

We removed our instruments under direct visualization, desufflating the abdomen completely. There was no bleeding from the trocar sites. The patient's bed was unflexed, and the fascial suture was tied. The skin and fascia were anesthetized with 0.25% Marcaine plain. The skin was closed with 4-0 Monocryl subcuticular stitch. Steri-Strips were applied. Sterile dressing was applied. The patient was transferred to the recovery room in stable and satisfactory condition.

Enter four diagnosis codes and one procedure code.

DX1

DX2

DX3

DX4

PR1

EXAM 3—SCENARIO 4

PREOPERATIVE DIAGNOSIS: Intraductal carcinoma in situ of the right breast

POSTOPERATIVE DIAGNOSIS: Intraductal carcinoma in situ of the right breast

PROCEDURE:

> Right needle-localized lumpectomy

> Axillary sampling

ANESTHESIA: General endotracheal

ESTIMATED BLOOD LOSS: Minimal

FLUIDS: 1,000 cc

DISPOSITION: To recovery room

INDICATIONS: The patient is a 71-year-old female who was noted to have abnormal calcifications at roughly the 6 o'clock position of the areola. These were biopsied and found to be intraductal carcinoma in situ. She was inclined to proceed with needle-localized lumpectomy. The risks of bleeding, infection, poor wound healing, and unappealing cosmetics were discussed. The possibility we could find invasive carcinoma was also discussed. The need for postoperative radiation therapy was also discussed. She was well aware of the possibility of positive margins that would lead to further surgery or a mastectomy.

PROCEDURE: The patient was initially taken to the Center for Breast Diagnosis, where Dr. X placed a needle at the inferior aspect of the breast.

The patient was then taken to the operating room. General anesthesia was administered. SCDs were placed. A curvilinear incision was made on the inferior aspect of the areola. This was taken down to the subcutaneous tissue. Flaps were raised in each direction for approximately 2 cm and taken down to the chest wall. A long stitch was placed medially, a short stitch superiorly.

The specimen was then removed. The cavity was then thoroughly irrigated; .25% Marcaine was used for local anesthesia. A sampling of axillary lymph nodes were removed.

The subcutaneous tissue was then approximated using 3-0 Monocryl. The skin was approximated using 4-0 Monocryl in a running subcuticular fashion. A sterile dressing was then applied.

The patient tolerated the procedure well and was taken to the recovery room. The operative findings were discussed with her husband and daughter.

Enter one diagnosis code and one procedure code.

DX1

PR1

EXAM 3—SCENARIO 5

ALLERGY INJECTIONS

DATE: 2/13/XX

LOCATION: Physician's office

NOTES: This 10-year-old male child presents to the physician's office to receive three allergy injections. He had been previously seen for repeated bouts of tonsillitis and sinus infections. The physician recommended allergy testing, which has been done and the results of the tests showed a need for three injections to be administered on a weekly basis because patient was found to be allergic to animal dander, pollen, grain, ragweed, and primrose. The child comes to the office today to receive the first series of his injections.

Enter two diagnosis codes and one procedure code.

DX1 [   ]

DX2 [   ]

PR1 [   ]

EXAM 3—SCENARIO 6

CARDIAC CATHETERIZATION PROCEDURE

DATE: 2/24/XX

LOCATION: Cath Lab

NOTES: This 72-year-old male patient presents today for cardiac catheterization following a week of testing for suspected cardiac problems. The patient was diagnosed with arteriosclerotic coronary artery heart disease. The physician performed a right and left heart catheterization including intraprocedural injection for left ventriculography.

Enter one diagnosis code and one procedure code.

DX1

PR1

EXAM 3—SCENARIO 7

DATE OF OPERATION: 10/26/20XX

PREOPERATIVE DIAGNOSIS: Hypertrophic pyloric stenosis

POSTOPERATIVE DIAGNOSES: Hypertrophic pyloric stenosis; thrombosed accessory spleen

OPERATION:

1. Laparoscopic pyloromyotomy

2. Excision of thrombosed accessory spleen

ANESTHESIA: General

INDICATIONS FOR SURGERY: Patient is a 4-week-old boy with a 1-week history of progressive projectile vomiting. Patient was brought to the emergency department, where he underwent ultrasound evaluation. Ultrasound findings revealed a pyloric channel of 15 mm in length with a wall thickness of 3.8 mm, consistent with hypertrophic pyloric stenosis. Electrolytes were found to be within reasonable range. Patient is brought to the operating room for pyloromyotomy.

FINDINGS: Moderately hypertrophied pylorus. No evidence of mucosal perforation. There was a 1 cm × 2 cm dark purple mass on the omentum, consistent with a thrombosed accessory spleen. This was excised without difficulty and sent for pathologic evaluation.

PROCEDURE: After informed consent was obtained, the patient was brought to the operating suite and placed in supine position. After adequate endotracheal anesthesia had been administered, his stomach was decompressed and his bladder was emptied, and his abdomen was prepared and draped in the usual sterile fashion. After infiltration with a local anesthetic, the base of the umbilicus was everted and a vertical 5-mm incision was made. A Veress needle was introduced, and pneumoperitoneum was established to 8 mm Hg pressure at 1 L/minute flow. The Veress needle was then replaced with a radially expandable 5-mm trocar. Laparoscope was introduced and confirmed good placement. Under laparoscopic visualization, stab incisions were made in the right upper quadrant and left upper quadrant. In the right upper quadrant, a pyloric grasper was introduced and in the left upper quadrant, the Arthro blade was introduced. Examination revealed a 1 cm × 2 cm dark purple mass attached to the omentum near the spleen. This was separate from the spleen. He had a normal-appearing lobulated spleen in the left upper quadrant. This mass was consistent with a thrombosed accessory spleen. Following the stomach distally, the pyloric channel was identified. This was moderately hypertrophied, consistent with the ultrasound diagnosis. While the pylorus was stabilized, the Arthro blade was extruded approximately 2 mm and used to incise the pylorus. The blade was then retracted, and the blunt tip was used to initiate the pyloromyotomy.

This then was replaced with a pyloric spreader, which was used to complete the pyloromyotomy. The mucosa was seen bulging without evidence of mucosal perforation. The pyloromyotomy was extended onto the antrum of the stomach. After there was good bulge of the mucosa, and the superior and inferior edges of the cut pylorus were independently mobile, the duodenum was occluded, and 40 cc of air was inflated into the stomach by the anesthesiologist. This revealed no evidence of a mucosal perforation. The stomach was then decompressed.

The laparoscope was removed and a 5-mm trocar was placed in the right upper quadrant incision site. Laparoscope confirmed good placement. The umbilical trocar was removed, and the umbilical incision was slightly extended to allow placement of an Endo catch bag. Prior to the introduction of the Endo catch bag, the lesion on the omentum was dissected free using electrocautery. There was good hemostasis. The Endo catch bag was then introduced through the umbilical trocar site and was used to retrieve the lesion without spillage or contamination. On palpation, this was soft but solid, consistent with a thrombosed accessory spleen. This was sent for pathologic review.

EXAM 3—SCENARIO 7 (*continued*)

Reexamination of the intraperitoneal cavity revealed good hemostasis. All instruments and trocars were removed, and the pneumoperitoneum was deflated. The fascia of the right upper quadrant trocar site and the umbilical trocar site were closed with 2-0 Vicryl in figure-of-8 stitch fashion. The umbilical skin incision was closed with 5-0 plain gut in interrupted stitch fashion. The other upper quadrant incisions were closed with Monocryl in subcuticular running stitch fashion. All incisions were cleaned and infiltrated with a local anesthetic. The umbilical trocar site was dressed with sterile gauze and Tegaderm. The other incisions were dressed with Steri-Strips. The patient tolerated the procedure well, was extubated, and then returned to the recovery room in stable condition.

PATHOLOGY REPORT

CLINICAL INFORMATION

PROCEDURE: Laparoscopic pyloromyotomy

PREOPERATIVE DIAGNOSIS: Pyloric stenosis (thrombosed accessory spleen)

CLINICAL HISTORY: Not given

GROSS DESCRIPTION:

Received fresh for routine examination designated R/O ACCESSORY SPLEEN is a 0.6 g, 1.1 cm × 1.0 cm × 0.5 cm, red-brown nodule with external smooth, glistening surface. The specimen is bisected and submitted entirely in one cassette.

MICROSCOPIC DESCRIPTION:

Sections through the accessory spleen revealed subcapsular markedly congested splenic sinusoids with minimal periarteriolar lymphocytic aggregates. Centrally the splenic tissue displays marked congestion and hemorrhage with loss of the sinusoidal pattern. Instead the parenchyma is largely replaced by capillaries with an intervening loose fibrin meshwork. At the periphery the hilum of the accessory spleen contains an extensive neutrophilic infiltrate. Scattered calcified nodules are noted within the splenic parenchyma.

DIAGNOSIS:

ABDOMINAL NODULE, EXCISION: ACCESSORY SPLEEN WITH CONGESTION AND HEMORRHAGE

Enter two diagnosis codes and two procedure codes.

DX1

DX2

PR1

PR2

EXAM 3—SCENARIO 8

REASON FOR VISIT: Left leg pain

HISTORY OF PRESENT ILLNESS: This is an 80-year-old diabetic resident at Nursing Manor. Patient has had this open wound in her left lower leg being dressed by nursing home staff twice a week. It has continued to get smaller, although for the past 5 days, she started having pain in the left leg that will start at the open wound and shoot all the way up to her hip. She has no fever or chills. Blood sugars are checking "normal" running around 114–120.

PHYSICAL EXAMINATION: Weight: 202; blood pressure: 130/58
This is an 80-year-old in no acute distress.

EXTREMITIES: Examination of her left leg shows no new swelling. There is some mild erythema around the open wound with some yellow exudate.

IMPRESSION:

1. Cellulitis, left leg

2. Diabetic peripheral vascular disease

PLAN: The patient was given 1 g of Rocephin IV push today in the office. Continue the dressings per Nursing Manor staff nurses. She may continue her pain medicine as needed. Recheck as needed.

HISTORY: Expanded problem

EXAMINATION: Expanded problem

MEDICAL DECISION-MAKING: Moderate

Enter two diagnosis codes and six procedure codes.

DX1

DX2

PR1

PR2

PR3

PR4

PR5

PR6

EXAM 4

For the following questions, choose the best answer. A blank answer sheet for these multiple-choice questions can be found on page 172.

Domain 1	*Diagnosis Coding*

1. This elderly female patient was examined today in the physician's office for the administration of her first radiation treatment for glioblastoma multiforme, which was recently diagnosed. The diagnosis was listed as "Radiotherapy for management of glioblastoma multiforme in her right occipital lobe." How is this coded?

Z51.0	Encounter for antineoplastic radiation therapy
Z51.11	Encounter for antineoplastic chemotherapy
C71.4	Malignant neoplasm of occipital lobe
C71.9	Malignant neoplasm of brain, unspecified

   a. Z51.0, C71.4

   b. Z51.11, C71.4

   c. Z51.0, C71.9

   d. Z51.11, C71.9

2. The patient with documented paranoid alcoholic psychosis is seen in the physician's office for a follow-up visit. Upon questioning, the patient reluctantly admits to experiencing some delusions and to an intake of large amounts of alcohol on a continuous basis. The physician schedules another appointment for the patient in one month and prescribes medicine for the diagnosis of delusions. How should this be coded?

F10.251	Alcohol dependence with alcohol-induced psychotic disorder with hallucinations
F10.229	Alcohol dependence with intoxication, unspecified
F10.250	Alcohol dependence with alcohol-induced psychotic disorder with delusions
F10.129	Alcohol abuse with intoxication, unspecified

   a. F10.251

   b. F10.250

   c. F10.229

   d. F10.129

3. An 84-year-old female is seen in the hematologist's office for pernicious anemia that has been recently diagnosed. This patient is also known to have agammaglobulinemia, a frequent occurrence in patients with pernicious anemia. This patient is also being treated for chronic atrophic gastritis, another condition associated with her anemia. She is being treated with medications for these conditions and will return to the hematologist's office in two months. What is the correct code assignment for this case?

D80.1	Nonfamilial hypogammaglobulinemia
D51.0	Vitamin B12 deficiency anemia due to intrinsic factor deficiency
D53.9	Nutritional anemia, unspecified
D53.0	Protein deficiency anemia
K29.40	Chronic atrophic gastritis without bleeding
K29.41	Chronic atrophic gastritis with bleeding
K29.00	Acute gastritis without bleeding

   a. D53.0, D80.1, K29.41

   b. D51.0, D80.1, K29.40

   c. D53.0, D80.1

   d. D53.9, D80.1, K29.00

4. Which of the following conditions is *not* considered a sequela of an injury?

   a. Paralysis of the right wrist due to previous laceration of right radial nerve

   b. Cellulitis in an open wound

   c. Nonunion fracture

   d. Posttraumatic scars due to old burn

5. A 20-year-old college student is seen in the health clinic with fever, malaise, myalgia, and anorexia. The physician documents clinical signs of swelling of both sides of the patient's face. Final diagnosis was listed as infectious parotitis. Which of the following would be reported?

   a. B26.9

   b. B26.9, R50.9, R53.81, R63.0, R59.0

   c. B26.89, R50.9, R53.81, R63.0, R59.0

   d. K11.20

6. A patient presents to the ED with hematuria. The patient admits to taking a combination of Coumadin and over-the-counter Alka-Seltzer for nasal congestion. The physician had not prescribed the Alka-Seltzer. The patient subsequently noticed blood in her urine. Which of the following would be reported?

   a. T45.511A, T39.011A

   b. T45.515A, T39.015A, R31.9

   c. T45.511A, T39.011A, R31.9

   d. T45.515A, T39.015A, R31.0

7. When coding sepsis and severe sepsis, which code should be sequenced first?

    a. Code for the postprocedural infection.

    b. Code for SIRS of a noninfectious origin.

    c. Code for the associated organ dysfunction(s).

    d. Code for the systemic infection.

8. The patient is a 57-year-old male who comes to the emergency department with severe abdominal pain. An acute gastric ulcer was identified following testing. There was no sign of malignancy or bleeding. The patient was placed on a special diet and discharged home. Which code is assigned?

    a. K25.7, Chronic gastric ulcer without hemorrhage or perforation

    b. K25.3, Acute gastric ulcer without hemorrhage or perforation

    c. K25.4, Chronic or unspecified gastric ulcer with hemorrhage

    d. K25.0, Acute gastric ulcer with hemorrhage

9. The patient is admitted with mild-stage pseudoexfoliation glaucoma of the right eye and moderate-stage low tension glaucoma of the left eye. What is the correct diagnosis code assignment for the physician's services?

H40.141	Capsular glaucoma with pseudoexfoliation of lens, right eye
H40.122	Low tension glaucoma, left eye
H40.143	Capsular glaucoma with pseudoexfoliation of lens, bilateral
	One of the following 7th characters is to be assigned to designate the stage of glaucoma
	0 stage unspecified
	1 mild stage
	2 moderate stage
	3 severe stage
	4 indeterminate stage

    a. H40.1432

    b. H40.1412, H40.1222

    c. H40.1411, H40.1222

    d. H40.1430

10. In which of the following situations would a code from category G89, Pain, NEC, be appropriate?

    a. The patient is having severe pain due to migraines.

    b. The patient is diagnosed with chest pain.

    c. The patient with lung cancer seeks medical care for neoplasm-related pain.

    d. The patient is seen in the ED with severe generalized abdominal pain.

11. The patient is admitted with metastatic carcinoma of the pancreas and omentum. How would the diagnoses for the physician services following admission be reported?

> | C48.1 | Malignant neoplasm of the specified parts of peritoneum |
> | C25.8 | Malignant neoplasm of overlapping sites of pancreas |
> | C25.9 | Malignant neoplasm of pancreas, unspecified |
> | C78.6 | Secondary malignant neoplasm of retroperitoneum and peritoneum |
> | C78.89 | Secondary malignant neoplasm of other digestive organs |
> | C80.1 | Malignant (primary) neoplasm, unspecified |

    a. C78.6, C78.89, C80.1

    b. C48.1, C25.9

    c. C78.6, C78.89

    d. C25.8, C25.9, C80.1

12. If there is a diagnosis of metastatic carcinoma of the lung, primary site was breast, but a mastectomy was done six years ago, then what is the reason for an encounter today?

    a. Metastatic carcinoma of the lung

    b. Carcinoma of the breast

    c. History of malignant neoplasm of the breast

    d. Status post mastectomy

13. The patient was admitted for elective cataract surgery that was successfully carried out. As the patient was preparing for discharge, she felt faint and weak and her blood pressure was quite low. It was determined that she should be admitted to the hospital for monitoring and treatment of the low blood pressure. The next day the patient was feeling much better and was discharged. The final diagnosis was orthostatic hypotension. What would be reported as the principal diagnosis for the hospital admission?

    a. Complication of cataract surgery

    b. Low blood pressure

    c. Orthostatic hypotension

    d. Weakness

14. The patient is a 79-year-old male who is being seen in the physician's office for follow-up of his condition and medication renewals. This patient has congestive heart failure resulting from his malignant hypertension, stage 3 chronic kidney disease and type 2 diabetes with polyneuropathy. The patient has been a diabetic for many years. How is this coded?

I13.0	Hypertensive heart and chronic kidney disease with heart failure and stage 1 through stage 4 chronic kidney disease, or unspecified chronic kidney disease
I13.10	Hypertensive heart and chronic kidney disease without heart failure, with stage 1 through stage 4 chronic kidney disease, or unspecified chronic kidney disease
I13.11	Hypertensive heart and chronic kidney disease without heart failure, with stage 5 chronic kidney disease or end stage renal disease
I50.9	Heart failure, unspecified
N17.9	Acute kidney failure, unspecified
N18.3	Chronic kidney disease, stage 3 unspecified
E11.42	Type 2 diabetes mellitus with diabetic polyneuropathy
E10.42	Type 1 diabetes mellitus with diabetic polyneuropathy

   a. I13.0, I50.9, N18.30, E11.42

   b. I13.10, I50.9, N18.30, E10.42

   c. I13.11, I50.9, N17.9, E11.42

   d. I13.0, N18.30, E11.42

15. The health record documentation states that the patient is treated in the ED in a coma due to accidental poisoning due to codeine. How would this ED encounter be coded?

T40.2X3X	Poisoning by other opioids, assault
R40.20	Unspecified coma
T40.2X1X	Poisoning by other opioids, accidental (unintentional)
T40.2X2X	Poisoning by other opioids, intentional self-harm
T40.2X5X	Adverse effect of other opioids
	Seventh character:
	A initial encounter
	D subsequent encounter
	S sequela

   a. T40.2X1A, R40.20

   b. T40.2X3D

   c. T40.2X1A, T40.2X5A

   d. T40.2X2D

16. The patient visits her OB/GYN physician at 29 weeks for a visit to monitor her benign essential hypertension, which she has had for several years now. How would this visit be coded?

   a. O10.013

   b. O10.013, Z3A.29

   c. I10, O10.013

   d. O16.3, Z3A.29

17. The excised diameter of a lesion means the measurement of:

    a. The largest lesion diameter

    b. The largest lesion diameter and the measurement of one margin

    c. The largest lesion diameter and the measurement of both margins

    d. The lesion length and width added together and the measurement of the margin

18. The patient undergoes a left heart catheterization and a left ventricular angiography using percutaneous femoral access. How is this procedure coded?

    a. 93452, Left heart catheterization including intraprocedural injection(s) for left ventriculography, imaging supervision and interpretation, when performed

    b. 93453, Combined right and left heart catheterization including intraprocedural injection(s) for left ventriculography, imaging supervision and interpretation, when performed

    c. 93458, Catheter placement in coronary artery(s) for coronary angiography, including intraprocedural injection(s) for coronary angiography, imaging supervision and interpretation; with left heart catheterization including intraprocedural injection(s) for left ventriculography, when performed

    d. 93460, Catheter placement in coronary artery(s) for coronary angiography, including intraprocedural injection(s) for coronary angiography, imaging supervision and interpretation; with right and left heart catheterization including intraprocedural injection(s) for left ventriculography, when performed

19. The patient undergoes an arthroscopic debridement of the articular cartilage and removal of meniscus in the lateral compartment of the right knee. How is this procedure coded?

29870	Arthroscopy, knee, diagnostic, with or without synovial biopsy (separate procedure)
29877	Arthroscopy, knee, surgical; debridement/shaving of articular cartilage (chondroplasty)
29881	with meniscectomy (medial OR lateral, including any meniscal shaving) including debridement/shaving of articular cartilage (chondroplasty), same or separate compartment(s), when performed
29882	with meniscus repair (medial OR lateral)

    a. 29881

    b. 29877, 29881

    c. 29877, 29882

    d. 29870, 29877, 29881

20. The physician replaces atrial and ventricular leads of a pacing cardioverter-defibrillator transvenously. The cardioverter-defibrillator was placed one year ago, and the battery remains intact. How is this coded?

    a. 33212, 33217, 33244

    b. 33215, 33215

    c. 33217, 33244

    d. 33218, 33218

21. The surgeon makes a burr hole in the skull over the cerebrum, based on stereotactic CT guidance, and aspirates a brain abscess via a needle. What is the correct code assignment for this case?

    a. 61140, 61782

    b. 61150, 61781

    c. 61156, 61781

    d. 61320, 61796

22. A patient with sick sinus syndrome has a leadless intraventricular pacemaker inserted along with initial interrogation and evaluation of the device. How is this coded?

    a. 33207

    b. 33207, 93289

    c. 33274

    d. 33274, 33275

23. The surgeon performs a laparoscopic myomectomy with removal of seven intramural myomas weighing 230 grams. What is the correct code assignment for this procedure?

    a. 58140

    b. 58146

    c. 58545

    d. 58546

24. The patient is the victim of blunt force abdominal trauma. The surgeon repairs the portion of the ruptured spleen that is salvageable and performs a partial splenectomy. What is the correct code assignment for these procedures?

    a. 38101

    b. 38115

    c. 38120

    d. 38129

25. The patient received a living, related donor renal transplant with removal of left kidney. Venous, arterial, and ureteral anastomoses were completed. The patient's peritoneal dialysis catheter was also removed. Backbench work was performed by a different surgeon. What is the correct code assignment for this case?

    a. 50365, 49422

    b. 50360, 49422

    c. 50365, 49429

    d. 50340, 50360, 50700, 35221, 49402

26. What information is needed to correctly assign a CPT emergency department evaluation and management code?

    a. Whether the patient is new or established to the emergency department physician

    b. How much time the physician spent with the patient

    c. What was the level of history, examination, and medical decision-making

    d. Whether the physician is an employee of the hospital

27. After comparing this patient encounter summary and the progress note, where does the coding manager find that education is needed?

Progress Note for 5-1-20XX

> S   This 10-year-old fell on the playground, cutting his right hand.
>
> O   There is a superficial palmar laceration measuring 2.0 cm.
>
> A   2.0 cm palmar laceration, washed with Betadine, anesthetized with 1% lidocaine and closed with one simple stitch of 5-0 nylon. Triple antibiotic ointment applied.
>
> P   Suture removal in one week.

Patient Encounter Summary:

Date	CPT Code	Code Description	Diagnosis	Diagnosis Description
5-1-20XX	13131	Repair, complex, forehead, cheeks, chin, mouth, neck, axillae, genitalia, hands and/or feet; 1.1 cm to 2.5 cm	S61.411A	Laceration without foreign body of right hand, initial encounter
5-1-20XX	99212	Office or other outpatient visit for the evaluation and management of an established patient, which requires a medically appropriate history and/or examination and straightforward medical decision making	S61.411A	Laceration without foreign body of right hand, initial encounter

a. A higher level of office visit should have been coded.

b. Modifier 59 should have been added to the office visit.

c. The documentation does not support the codes assigned.

d. The local anesthetic should have been coded.

28. The physician provides 115 minutes of critical care to the patient and documents the time in the record. How is this service coded?

> 99291   Critical care, evaluation and management of the critically ill or critically injured patient; first 30–74 minutes
>
> 99292   each additional 30 minutes (List separately in addition to code for primary service)

a. 99291

b. 99291, 99292

c. 99291, 99292, 99292

d. 99291, 99292, 99292, 99292

29. A new physician submits four encounters from his first day in clinic. They were all completed incorrectly because a procedure was performed with an E/M visit. What is the best action for the coding professional to take to resolve the situation for the future?

    a. Recode the charges and then submit them.

    b. Educate the physician about the appropriate use of modifier 25 and the surgical package reporting guidelines.

    c. Ask the office manager to inform the physician that procedures are not performed in the office setting.

    d. Refuse to process charges until the physician receives formal training.

30. A patient presents for a follow-up with her endocrinologist. The physician gives the patient a diagnosis of thyroid cancer. The physician documents a problem-focused history and exam, which takes only five minutes. From there, the physician documents that he spent the next 40 minutes discussing the patient's prognosis, options, answering questions, and making referrals for further care. How would this visit be coded?

    a. 99212

    b. 99215

    c. 99241

    d. 99243

31. The patient presents for a diagnostic colonoscopy. Due to poor preparation, the physician is not able to advance the scope beyond the splenic flexure. How is this service coded?

45330	Sigmoidoscopy, flexible; diagnostic, including collection of specimen(s) by brushing or washing, when performed (separate procedure)
45378	Colonoscopy, flexible; diagnostic, including collection of specimen(s) by brushing or washing, when performed (separate procedure)
-22	Increased procedural services
-52	Reduced services
-53	Discontinued procedure

    a. 45378-52

    b. 45378-53

    c. 45330

    d. 45330-22

32. The physician performs a procedure that cannot be described with a regular code in CPT, so an unlisted code is assigned. The physician wants modifier 22 applied to the code. What is the best action for the coding professional to take?

    a. Apply modifier 22 to the unlisted code as requested by the physician.

    b. Explain to the physician that modifiers cannot be used on unlisted codes.

    c. Submit a different CPT code that describes a lesser procedure and add modifier 22.

    d. Submit a different CPT code that describes a more extensive procedure and add modifier 52.

33. The following is a summary of visits for John Smith on November 2:

> 9:30 a.m.   Seen by Dr. X for asthma, requiring nebulizer treatment and medication
> 3:30 p.m.   Seen by Dr. X again for worsening asthma, requiring another nebulizer treatment and more medication

To help ensure payment, which of the following modifiers should be reported by Dr. X for the services provided at 3:30 p.m.?

a. -51, Multiple procedures

b. -58, Staged or related procedure or service by the same physician or other qualified health care professional during the postoperative period

c. -76, Repeat procedure or service by same physician or other qualified health care professional

d. -77, Repeat procedure by another physician or other qualified health care professional

34. A patient undergoes open treatment of a femoral fracture following a car accident. Two weeks later, the patient falls out of his wheelchair and must return to the operating room for closed treatment of a humeral shaft fracture. The same physician performs both procedures. What modifier must be appended to the CPT code for the second procedure?

a. -76

b. -77

c. -78

d. -79

35. All of the following information is needed to correctly code skin grafts *except:*

a. Size of the defect

b. Location of the donor site

c. Type of graft used

d. Location of the defect

36. The patient presents to the physician's office with fever and chills and is diagnosed with pneumonia. The physician administers 600 mg of Rocephin, IV over 1 hour and 31 minutes. In addition to the E/M code, how are these services coded?

> J0696   Injection, ceftriaxone sodium, per 250 mg
> 96365   Intravenous infusion, for therapy, prophylaxis, or diagnosis (specify substance or drug); initial, up to 1 hour
> 96366   each additional hour (List separately in addition to code for primary procedure.)
> 96374   Therapeutic, prophylactic, or diagnostic injection (specify substance or drug); intravenous push, single or initial substance/drug

a. 96374, J0696

b. 96365, J0696 ×2

c. 96365, 96366, J0696

d. 96365, 96366, J0696 ×3

37. When should the coding professional assign a code for a cast application?

    a. When applying a removable splint

    b. When revising a cast the patient is now wearing

    c. When a fracture treatment has been provided

    d. When applying a replacement cast during or after the period of normal follow-up care

38. The patient undergoes a proctosigmoidoscopy, a sigmoidoscopy with biopsy, and a colonoscopy during the same operative session. What is the correct coding assignment for these services?

45300	Proctosigmoidoscopy, rigid; diagnostic, with or without collection of specimen(s) by brushing or washing (separate procedure)
45305	with biopsy, single or multiple
45330	Sigmoidoscopy, flexible; diagnostic, including collection of specimen(s) by brushing or washing, when performed (separate procedure)
45331	with biopsy, single or multiple
45378	Colonoscopy, flexible; diagnostic, including collection of specimen(s) by brushing or washing, when performed (separate procedure)
45380	with biopsy, single or multiple

    a. 45378

    b. 45380

    c. 45300, 45331, 45378

    d. 45305, 45331, 45380

39. On the third day of the patient's inpatient stay, the physician visits with the patient for 20 minutes and documents a problem-focused interval history, a problem-focused exam, and medical decision-making of low complexity. Which code would be used to report this service?

    a. 99213

    b. 99221

    c. 99231

    d. 99251

40. The patient had a total abdominal hysterectomy with bilateral salpingo-oophorectomy. The coding professional selected the following codes to report:

58150	Total abdominal hysterectomy (corpus and cervix), with or without removal of tube(s), with or without removal of ovary(s)
58700	Salpingectomy, complete or partial, unilateral or bilateral (separate procedure)

What error has the coding professional made by using these codes?

    a. Maximizing

    b. Upcoding

    c. Unbundling

    d. Optimizing

41. A total laparoscopic-assisted vaginal hysterectomy with bilateral salpingo-oophorectomy is performed. The uterus was greater than 250 grams. How is this coded?

    a. 58541

    b. 58553, 58720

    c. 58554

    d. 58572

42. The physician performing the procedure also provides anesthesia for the procedure. What is the National Correct Coding Initiative (NCCI) policy in this situation?

    a. The physician may report both the procedure and the anesthesia service.

    b. The anesthesia service may not be reported in any circumstance.

    c. The anesthesia service may only be reported if provided by a second provider.

    d. They physician may unbundle components of the anesthesia and report each one separately with modifier 59.

43. A patient presents to her primary care physician's office for her quarterly visit. The physician performs a medically appropriate history and exam. He reviews her CMP and Hemoglobin A1C, both of which are normal. He also orders thyroid function studies. He refills her medications to treat her hypertension, diabetes, and anxiety. A follow-up appointment is scheduled in three months. How would this visit be coded?

99203	Office or other outpatient visit for the evaluation and management of a new patient, which requires a medically appropriate history and/or examination and low level of medical decision making
99204	Office or other outpatient visit for the evaluation and management of a new patient, which requires a medically appropriate history and/or examination and moderate level of medical decision making
99213	Office or other outpatient visit for the evaluation and management of an established patient, which requires a medically appropriate history and/or examination and low level of medical decision making
99214	Office or other outpatient visit for the evaluation and management of an established patient, which requires a medically appropriate history and/or examination and moderate level of medical decision making

    a. 99203

    b. 99204

    c. 99213

    d. 99214

44. A physician documents total time spent with his established patient in the office was one hour and twenty minutes. How would this visit be coded?

> | 99205 | Office or other outpatient visit for the evaluation and management of a new patient, which requires a medically appropriate history and/or examination and high level of medical decision making. When using time for code selection, 60–74 minutes of total time is spent on the date of the encounter. |
> | 99215 | Office or other outpatient visit for the evaluation and management of an established patient, which requires a medically appropriate history and/or examination and high level of medical decision making. When using time for code selection, 40–54 minutes of total time is spent on the date of the encounter. |
> | +99417 | Prolonged office or other outpatient evaluation and management service(s) beyond the minimum required time of the primary procedure which has been selected using total time, requiring total time with or without direct patient contact beyond the usual service, on the date of the primary service, each 15 minutes of total time. |

a. 99205

b. 99205, 99417

c. 99215

d. 99215, 99417, 99417

45. A patient diagnosed with incomplete abortion at 15 weeks undergoes a D&C. How would this procedure be coded?

> | 57520 | Conization of cervix, with or without fulguration, with or without dilation and curettage, with or without repair; cold knife or laser |
> | 58120 | Dilation and curettage, diagnostic and/or therapeutic (nonobstetrical) |
> | 59812 | Treatment of incomplete abortion, any trimester, completed surgically |
> | 59840 | Induced abortion, by dilation and curettage |

a. 57520

b. 58120

c. 59812

d. 59840

46. The physician performs a core needle biopsy of a lesion of the epididymis. How would this be coded?

> | 10021 | Fine needle aspiration biopsy, without imaging guidance; first lesion |
> | 54800 | Biopsy of epididymis, needle |
> | 54830 | Excision of local lesion of epididymis |

a. 10021

b. 54800

c. 54830

d. 54830, 10021

47. The physician performs a bilateral myringotomy with insertion of ventilating tubes under general anesthesia. How would this be coded?

> 69420   Myringotomy including aspiration and/or eustachian tube inflation
> 69436   Tympanostomy (requiring insertion of ventilating tube), general anesthesia
> -50   Bilateral Procedure

    a. 69420-50
    b. 69420, 69420
    c. 69436-50
    d. 69436, 69436

48. A patient was admitted to the hospital as an inpatient, immediately following an outpatient consultation at the physician's office. The physician documented a comprehensive history, a comprehensive exam, and medical decision-making of moderate complexity. Later that same day, the physician discharged the patient. How would these services be coded by the physician?

> 99222   Initial hospital care, per day, for the evaluation and management of a patient, which requires these 3 key components: a comprehensive history; a comprehensive exam; and medical decision making of moderate complexity
> 99238   Hospital discharge day management; 30 minutes or less
> 99244   Office consultation for a new or established patient which requires these 3 components: a comprehensive history; a comprehensive examination; medical decision making of moderate complexity
> 99235   Observation or inpatient hospital care for the evaluation and management of a patient including admission and discharge on the same date, which requires 3 three key components: a comprehensive history; a comprehensive examination; and medical decision making of moderate complexity

    a. 99244, 99222, 99238
    b. 99222, 99238
    c. 99244, 99235
    d. 99235

Domain 3   *Research*

49. In which HCPCS category would the coding professional find temporary codes for screening cytopathology to code services provided to patients covered by Medicare?
    a. G0008–G9157
    b. J0120–J9999
    c. P2028–P9615
    d. Q0035–Q9983

50. A patient is evaluated by his family practitioner for acute chest pain. The physician documents as the final diagnosis chest pain due to probable gastric ulcer and a history of cholecystectomy. What should the coding professional report?

    a. Chest pain; gastric ulcer

    b. Gastric ulcer

    c. Chest pain

    d. Chest pain; history of cholecystectomy

51. An asymptomatic Medicare patient with a family history of colon cancer and a personal history of colon polyps undergoes an examination of the entire colon and the terminal ileum. What is the correct coding assignment for this procedure?

    a. G0104, Colorectal cancer screening, flexible sigmoidoscopy

    b. G0105, Colorectal cancer screening, colonoscopy on individual at high risk

    c. 45300, Proctosigmoidoscopy, rigid diagnostic, with or without collection of specimen(s) by brushing or washing (separate procedure)

    d. 45378, Colonoscopy, flexible; diagnostic, including collection of specimen(s) by brushing or washing, when performed (separate procedure)

52. A coding professional has a question about how to use a newly created ICD-10-CM code. What would be the best reference?

    a. *CPT Assistant*

    b. *Coding Clinic*

    c. Local coverage determinations (LCDs)

    d. Correct coding initiatives

53. All of the following are useful for establishing medical necessity and assuring appropriate reimbursement for services provided *except:*

    a. Local coverage determinations

    b. National coverage determinations

    c. Encoders and groupers

    d. Advanced Beneficiary Notice

54. The best way for a coding professional to avoid unbundling, is to consult:

    a. National Correct Coding Initiative (NCCI)

    b. National coverage determinations

    c. AHIMA practice briefs

    d. CPT changes

55. The physician sees a patient with documented colitis, enteritis, and diarrhea. Which of the following should the coding professional assign to this case?

    a. K52.9

    b. K52.9, R19.7

    c. A09, R19.7

    d. K52.9, A09, R19.7

56. In which of the following situations would a physician query be required?

    a. A routine preoperative chest x-ray on a 95-year-old patient reveals a collapsed vertebral body. The patient is being evaluated for pneumonia.

    b. In the absence of a cardiac problem an EKG on a 97-year-old shows cardiomegaly.

    c. The lab work shows low potassium level and the coding professional notes that the patient was given oral potassium.

    d. The physician documents gram-negative sepsis with no culture documented or symptoms noted.

57. Queries are appropriate for documentation that is not legible, complete, clear, consistent, precise, reliable, or timely. Documentation that does not contradict itself is deemed:

    a. Consistent

    b. Precise

    c. Reliable

    d. Complete

58. Which of the following is true about the goal of physician queries?

    a. To document the highest severity condition to increase reimbursement

    b. To prompt physicians to select higher-paying diagnoses

    c. To question the clinical expertise of the provider

    d. To achieve the greatest amount of specificity and accuracy

59. A 55-year-old morbidly obese female with familial hypercholesterolemia was seen in her physician's office for a follow-up visit. She has managed to control her condition with medication and was also counseled at this time to maintain her smoke-free status. An appointment was set up for a return visit in four months. What is the correct code assignment for this case?

E78.01	Familial hypercholesterolemia
E78.5	Hyperlipidemia, unspecified
E66.9	Obesity, unspecified
E66.01	Morbid (severe) obesity due to excess calories
E66.3	Overweight

    a. E78.01, E66.9

    b. E78.5, E66.3

    c. E78.01, E66.01

    d. E78.5, E66.9

60. A 12-year-old girl comes to the physician's office with her grandmother because of the following complaints: fever, discolored nasal discharge, puffy eyes, stuffy nose, and pain in the cheek areas. The physician examined her and confirmed her complaints. The physician also detected fluid in her sinuses. The physician diagnosed acute sinusitis in the maxillary and frontal sinuses and prescribed antibiotics and Tylenol. How is this coded?

J01.80	Other acute sinusitis
J01.90	Acute sinusitis, unspecified
J32.0	Chronic maxillary sinusitis
J32.9	Chronic sinusitis, unspecified

    a. J32.0, J01.80

    b. J01.90, J32.9

    c. J01.80, J32.0

    d. J01.80

61. When coding a colposcopy with LEEP, what type of documentation is most likely to affect code assignment?

    a. Was the examination performed under anesthesia?

    b. Was a conization performed?

    c. Did the pathology report show malignancy?

    d. Did the procedure include injection of dye or saline?

62. A six-year-old established patient is seen for a well-child check at her pediatrician's office. After completing and documenting the visit, the physician explains to the child's mother that it is time for the child's measles, mumps, rubella, and varicella vaccines. The physician counsels the mother, obtains consent, and administers the vaccine. Which CPT codes would be used to report this encounter?

    a. 99383, 90460, 90461, 90710

    b. 99383, 90471, 90472, 90710

    c. 99393, 90460, 90461 × 3, 90710

    d. 99393, 90471, 90472 × 3, 90710

63. Which of the following describes selecting diagnosis or procedure codes solely to increase reimbursement from third-party payers?

    a. Optimizing

    b. Maximization

    c. Unbundling

    d. Upcoding

64. Which of the following seeks the most accurate documentation, coded date, and resulting payment that the provider is legally entitled to receive?

    a. Optimization

    b. Maximization

    c. Upcoding

    d. Bundling

65. In order to use codes from the consultation subsection of CPT's evaluation and management codes:

    a. The patient being referred must have requested a second opinion.

    b. The consulting physician must document and sign a report stating his opinion and send it back to the referring physician.

    c. The consulting physician must document and sign that he or she is assuming care of the patient.

    d. The history and physical provided by the consulting physician must be dated and signed.

66. A one-year-old established patient presents to the pediatrician for a physical, MMR, and varicella vaccinations. After reviewing the following coding in an audit, what audit findings did the coding manager determine?

    Patient: Jane Doe
    DOB: 2-28-2010

Date of Service	CPT Code	Code Description	Diagnosis	Diagnosis Description
2-28-2011	99392	Periodic comprehensive preventive medicine reevaluation and management of an individual including an age and gender appropriate history, examination, counseling/anticipatory guidance/ risk factor reduction interventions, and the ordering of laboratory/ diagnostic procedures, established patient; early childhood (age 1 through 4 years)	Z00.129 Z23	Encounter for routine child health examination without abnormal findings Encounter for immunization
2-28-2011	90707	Measles, mumps and rubella virus vaccine (MMR), live, for subcutaneous use	Z00.129 Z23	Encounter for routine child health examination without abnormal findings Encounter for immunization
2-28-2011	90716	Varicella virus vaccine (VAR), live, for subcutaneous use	Z00.129 Z23	Encounter for routine child health examination, without abnormal findings Encounter for immunization

    a. The CPT code(s) are incorrect.

    b. The ICD-10-CM code(s) are incorrect.

    c. CPT code(s) are missing.

    d. The case is coded correctly.

67. The patient is admitted with shortness of breath and cough and is diagnosed with MRSA *Staphylococcus aureus* pneumonia. The physician also documents a MRSA colonization. Which of the following would be reported?

    a. J15.212, Z22.322

    b. J15.212

    c. J15.212, Z22.322, R06.02, R05.3

    d. J15.212, R06.02, R05.9

68. The term that refers to the degree to which the same results are achieved each time a health record is coded during a coding audit is:

    a. Validity

    b. Completeness

    c. Reliability

    d. Timeliness

69. Which of the following conditions would not be included in the CMS-HCC model?

    a. Acute respiratory infection

    b. Metastatic liver cancer

    c. Ischemic or unspecified stroke

    d. Lymphoma

70. There are several types of risk adjustment models that are used to risk-adjust healthcare data. Which of these is used in Medicare's Advantage C program?

    a. RxHCC

    b. HHS-HCC

    c. CMS-HCC

    d. 3M-APR-DRGs

71. The patient asked for and received a copy of the disclosures that were made of his PHI. He did not see his attending physician on the list and was concerned that the physician did not have the information. What is the patient told?

    a. The organization cannot release that information to the patient.

    b. Disclosures used for treatment are not recorded so that is why the physician's name does not appear on the list.

    c. The physician apparently never asked for the records.

    d. The patient should speak with his physician as to why the records were not requested.

72. According to HIPAA, policies and procedures necessary to ensure compliance with the privacy rules must be written and maintained for:

    a. 5 years

    b. 6 years

    c. 10 years

    d. Indefinitely

73. With regards to a breach, what number of patient records is considered a "significant threshold," requiring a covered entity to immediately report the breach to the secretary of HHS?

    a. 100

    b. 250

    c. 500

    d. 1,000

74. A pattern, practice, or specific activity that may indicate identity theft is a:

    a. Breach

    b. Legal health record

    c. Mitigation

    d. Red flag

75. After completing a quality audit on this patient encounter summary, what action should the coding supervisor take?

    Patient Encounter Summary
    Dr. Dunn, Primary Care
    Patient #784309

Date of Service	CPT Code	Code Description	Diagnosis	Charge
5/1/20XX	73610	Radiologic examination, ankle; complete, minimum of 3 views	M25.572	$76.00
5/1/20XX	27816	Closed treatment of trimalleolar ankle fracture; without manipulation	S82.852A	$249.00
5/1/20XX	Q4038	Cast supplies, short leg cast, adult (11 years +), fiberglass	S82.852A	$43.00
5/1/20XX	29405	Application of short leg cast (below knee to toes)	S82.852A	$65.00

    a. Clarify the fracture treatment with the physician.

    b. Instruct the physician about proper coding of cast applications.

    c. Instruct the physician to add an office visit.

    d. Query the physician about the correct diagnosis.

76. As office manager, you are planning an in-service presentation on documentation for critical care. You tell the nursing staff that the following must be included on the health record in order to bill properly:

    a. Place the critical care was offered

    b. Total nursing time that was spent with the patient

    c. Names of all physicians who provided critical care services at the same time

    d. Procedures that are not bundled into the critical care codes

77.

HCPCS CODE	Description	Work RVU	Nonfacility PE	Facility PE	MP RVU
53505	Repair of urethra injury	8.26	NA	4.99	0.99

Locality Name	20XX PW GPCI	20XX PE GPCI	20XX MP GPCI
ALABAMA	1.000	0.889	0.707

What would be the total RVUs for a physician who repaired a urethral injury for a patient in the local ED in Alabama?

a. 8.9599

b 14

c. 13.3960

d. 13.4

78.

HCPCS CODE	Description	Work RVU	Nonfacility PE	Facility PE	MP RVU
52317	Litholapaxy: crushing or fragmentation of calculus by any means in bladder and removal of fragments; simple or small (less than 2.5 cm)	6.71	17.48	2.55	.78

Locality Name	20XX PW GPCI	20XX PE GPCI	20XX MP GPCI
SAN DIEGO-CARLSBAD	1.032	1.130	0.607

Conversion Factor for 20XX: $36.88

How much would a physician be reimbursed in total by CMS and the patient for removing a bladder stone in her clinic in San Diego?

a. $1,001.31

b. $811.50

c. $379.11

d. $303.28

79. A physician initiates treatment and establishes a plan of care. The nurse practitioner (NP), who is trained in wound care, sees the patient weekly over the next 12 weeks to monitor and treat the wound. The physician is present, on site, during all of these monitoring/treating visits by the NP. The provider sees the patient every fourth visit, under a policy adopted by the practice. How would the billing personnel submit these claims?

a. The office visits with the NP would be billed under the NP's National Provider Identifier (NPI) and the visits with the physician under the physician's NPI.

b. All of the visits would be billed under the physician's NPI.

c. The visits by the NP would not be billed, but the office visit with the physician would be billed under the physician's NPI.

d. All of the visits would be billed under the NP's NPI.

80. A surgical patient has an established diagnosis and plan of care and is seen by the physician's assistant (PA) who identifies a new problem. The PA asks the surgeon, who is in the office, to see the patient. The surgeon evaluates the patient and initiates a course of treatment for the newly identified problem. How is this office visit billed?

    a. Both the PA and the surgeon can bill an office visit for this patient; modifier 51 is required.

    b. The office visit is billed under the surgeon's National Provider Identifier (NPI).

    c. The office visit is billed under the PA's NPI.

    d. Both the PA and the surgeon can bill an office visit for this patient; modifier 51 is not required.

81. Which of the following provides facilities and physicians with the circumstances under which a service, procedure, or supply is considered medically necessary within the jurisdiction of a particular MAC?

    a. National coverage determinations

    b. Local coverage determinations

    c. CMS transmittals

    d. National Correct Coding Initiative

82. Which of the following is not a type of claim denial?

    a. Clinical denial

    b. Administrative denial

    c. Clinical validation denial

    d. Ancillary service denial

83. Which government agency released the elements of an effective corporate compliance plan?

    a. OIG

    b. CMS

    c. Agency on Aging

    d. FBI

84. Which of the following statements is true about coding laterality in ICD-10-CM?

    a. Laterality assignment is based only on physician documentation.

    b. If the laterality is not stated, use the code for the patient's dominant side.

    c. Two codes are always needed to show laterality if the term *bilateral* is used.

    d. If there is conflicting documentation regarding the affected side, the patient's provider should be queried for clarification.

85. Which of the following cannot be coded based on documentation from someone other than the patient's provider?

    a. Body mass index

    b. Pressure ulcer stage

    c. Alcohol-related disorders

    d. Social determinants of health

86. Which of the following is true about coding conditions related to COVID-19?

    a. For asymptomatic individuals with actual exposure to COVID-19, assign code Z20.822, contact with and (suspected) exposure to COVID-19.

    b. For asymptomatic individuals with suspected exposure to COVID-19, do not assign code Z20.822, contact with and (suspected) exposure to COVID-19.

    c. For asymptomatic individuals who test positive for COVID-19, assign code Z20.822, contact with and (suspected) exposure to COVID-19.

    d. For patients with a history of COVID-19, continue to assign code U07.1, COVID-19.

Domain 5 *Revenue Cycle*

87. Which report contains a summary of all billing data entered for a physician's practice for one day, listing all vital pieces of data to be included on the billing form?

    a. Claim history

    b. Diagnosis distribution

    c. Charge summary report

    d. Frequency distribution

88. When a patient is covered by Medicare, which of the following services will be reimbursed?

    a. General health laboratory panel

    b. Consultation E/M codes

    c. A preventive medicine service at the start of coverage

    d. Certain transplant services such as pancreas and cornea

89. The greatest percent of claims denials occur due to errors in which of the revenue cycle processes:

    a. Charge capture

    b. Registration

    c. Claims submission

    d. Claims preparation

90. This information is published by the Medicare Administrative Contractors (MACs) to describe when and under what circumstances Medicare will cover a service in a distinct area:

    a. Local coverage determinations

    b. Medicare Claims Processing Manual

    c. CMS program transmittals

    d. National coverage determinations

91. The patient is seen at Wolf Place Physician Practice. The total charge for the visit is $300.00. The physician is a nonparticipating (non-PAR) physician who accepts assignment and the patient has met the deductible for 20XX. The Medicare fee schedule amount for the E/M code is $200.00. What is the amount that the federal government will reimburse the physician?

    a. $300.00

    b. $200.00

    c. $190.00

    d. $152.00

92. Medicare's resource-based relative value scale payment system is modified by a formula that includes time and base units for which type of provider?

    a. Nonphysician providers

    b. Physician assistants

    c. Anesthesiologists

    d. Nonparticipating physicians

93. Which of the following is *not* one of the more common forms of fraud and abuse?

    a. Falsifying medical necessity to justify payment

    b. Billing for services not furnished

    c. Misrepresenting the diagnosis to increase payment

    d. Failing to have a compliance officer in the facility

94. Screening for medical necessity is part of the _____ process in revenue cycle management.

    a. Preregistration

    b. Charge capture

    c. Claims submission

    d. Claims reconciliation

95. Which of the following would be helpful in finding information about medical necessity and documentation guidelines?

    a. OIG Work Plan

    b. National Correct Coding Initiative

    c. Local coverage determinations

    d. Medicare Claims Processing Manuals

96. Relative value units (RVUs) are adjusted to local costs through the geographic practice cost indices (GPCIs). Which RVUs are adjusted by the GPCIs?

    a. Work and Practice Expense

    b. Work and Malpractice

    c. Practice Expense and Malpractice

    d. Work, Practice Expense, and Malpractice

97. The physician performed a rigid bronchoscopy, diagnostic with a transbronchial lung biopsy of a single lobe, CPT code 31628. Which documentation would the coding professional most likely see on the record for this patient?

    a. Acute laryngopharyngitis (J06.0)

    b. Pulmonary edema due to chemicals, gases, fumes and vapors (J68.1)

    c. Malignant neoplasm of trachea (C33)

    d. Malignant neoplasm of middle lobe, bronchus or lung (C34.2)

Multiple Choice Exam 4 Answers

1.	26.	51.	76.
2.	27.	52.	77.
3.	28.	53.	78.
4.	29.	54.	79.
5.	30.	55.	80.
6.	31.	56.	81.
7.	32.	57.	82.
8.	33.	58.	83.
9.	34.	59.	84.
10.	35.	60.	85.
11.	36.	61.	86.
12.	37.	62.	87.
13.	38.	63.	88.
14.	39.	64.	89.
15.	40.	65.	90.
16.	41.	66.	91.
17.	42.	67.	92.
18.	43.	68.	93.
19.	44.	69.	94.
20.	45.	70.	95.
21.	46.	71.	96.
22.	47.	72.	97.
23.	48.	73.	
24.	49.	74.	
25.	50.	75.	

EXAM 4 MEDICAL SCENARIOS

EXAM 4—SCENARIO 1

HISTORY: Follow-up decompression laminectomy and extension of fusion lumbar spine L2 to sacrum performed 1 year ago. Patient generally doing pretty well with back, has achy back discomfort. Main problem is bilateral lateral hip pain. She has a previous diagnosis of trochanteric bursitis. She also describes triggering of her right middle finger with catching of the finger in flexion. The patient had a right knee replacement several years previously.

PHYSICAL EXAMINATION:

VITAL SIGNS: Blood pressure 137/77; Pulse 79; Temperature is 98.1

HEENT: Normal

CHEST: Clear

HEART: Normal sinus rhythm, no murmur

SPINE EXAMINATION: Reveals well-healed incision lumbar spine with minimal tenderness, no paravertebral spasm. Range of motion 80% of normal.

HIP EXAMINATION: Reveals full range of motion of hips bilaterally. There is exquisite tenderness over abductor insertion on greater trochanter.

HAND EXAMINATION: Reveals triggering of the right middle finger.

RADIOGRAPHS: Previous x-rays of lumbar spine reviewed showing excellent instrumented fusion L2 to sacrum with fusion consolidation. Extensive narrowing of the spine at the T3–T4 region.

IMPRESSION:

1. Stenosis in thoracic spinal area

2. Bilateral trochanteric bursitis

3. Right middle trigger finger

PLAN:

1. Trochanteric bursa is injected bilateral today under sterile conditions using 5 cc of Kenalog.

2. Right middle finger injected today with improvement with 0.5 cc of Kenalog.

3. Flexeril 10 mg p.o. t.i.d. p.r.n. Renew hydrocodone 5/500 1 p.o. q.6 h p.r.n. pain.

4. Consider surgery on stenosed thoracic region of the spine.

5. Return in 6 months' time for reevaluation.

MEDICAL DECISION-MAKING: Moderate level

TIME: 30 minutes spent with patient

Enter four diagnosis codes and five procedure codes.

DX1

DX2

DX3

DX4

PR1

PR2

PR3

PR4

PR5

EXAM 4—SCENARIO 2

CONSULT REQUESTED BY: Dr. A

HISTORY: The patient is a 33-year-old female who has had known gallstones and postprandial right upper quadrant and epigastric pain for the past 3 years. She describes the pain as intense gas pains. The pain radiates occasionally to her back. She notes that her pain is worse with fatty food. She has tried herbal remedies without success. She has no history of jaundice or pancreatitis. She has had no emergency department visits or hospitalizations for the pain. The pain is worsening, and the patient is sent here for evaluation and definitive diagnosis.

PAST MEDICAL HISTORY:

1. Iron deficiency anemia

PAST SURGICAL HISTORY: None

ALLERGIES: Penicillin

MEDICATIONS:

1. Multivitamins

2. Iron 65 mg, two daily

FAMILY HISTORY: The patient's paternal grandmother had breast cancer. Her paternal grandfather had colon cancer. Her maternal grandfather had lung cancer. Diabetes and hypertension also run in her family.

REVIEW OF SYSTEMS: A 14-point review of systems was completed by the patient today in the office. The patient reports weight gain as well as back pain. She denies any chest pain, shortness of breath, or dysuria. The remaining review of systems is negative.

SOCIAL HISTORY: The patient is married. She works as a managed care coordinator. She does not smoke. She drinks alcohol occasionally.

PHYSICAL EXAMINATION:

VITAL SIGNS: Weight 229.4 pounds; blood pressure 129/72; heart rate is 86; temperature 97.5

GENERAL: The patient is a pleasant female in no acute distress. Alert and oriented times three.

HEENT: There is no jaundice, thyroid masses, or cervical lymphadenopathy.

RESPIRATORY: Lung sounds are clear bilaterally

HEART: Regular rate and rhythm

ABDOMEN: Soft and nontender. There are no scars or hernias.

MUSCULOSKELETAL: Gait, strength, and muscle tone within normal limits

NEUROLOGIC: Cranial nerves II–XII are grossly intact

DATA: Abdominal ultrasound report shows the gallbladder was markedly contracted with multiple stones. The common bile duct measured 6 mm in diameter.

LABORATORY: Laboratory dated 11/22/20XX, bilirubin 0.2, AST 20, ALT 28, alkaline phosphatase 29, amylase 62, lipase 21

ASSESSMENT/PLAN: The patient is a 33-year-old otherwise healthy woman with classic symptoms of biliary colic. We had an extensive discussion with the patient in regard to the technical aspects of the laparoscopic cholecystectomy. We discussed the potential complications of the surgery that include but are not limited to: need to convert to open surgery, retained stone, bile duct injury, bleeding,

EXAM 4—SCENARIO 2 (*continued*)

infection, DVT, and pneumonia. All of her questions were answered to her satisfaction. Because of the frequency of her pain, she is eager to proceed with surgery. We have tentatively scheduled her surgery for December 13th. If she develops any questions or concerns, she should call the office.

CC: Dr. A

HISTORY: Comprehensive

EXAMINATION: Comprehensive

MEDICAL DECISION-MAKING: Moderate

Enter one diagnosis code and one procedure code.

DX1

PR1

EXAM 4—SCENARIO 3

PREOPERATIVE DIAGNOSIS: Right carotid stenosis

POSTOPERATIVE DIAGNOSIS: Right carotid stenosis

PROCEDURE: Right carotid endarterectomy

INDICATION: This patient is a 53-year-old male who was recently hospitalized. During the course of his workup, he was noted to have a right carotid stenosis. This was asymptomatic. Angiography confirmed the finding, and it appeared to be approximately 80% stenosis in the right internal carotid artery. The opposite carotid artery is in good condition. The patient was carefully advised about the risks, benefits, and alternatives for asymptomatic carotid stenosis, including the magnitude of reduction of stroke risk in comparison with the actual stroke risk without surgery. The patient understood that this is a purely prophylactic procedure that could cause stroke as a risk and other complications such as tongue paralysis, lower right lip paralysis, numbness in the neck, bleeding, infection, paralysis, and death. He understands the above and requested that surgery be performed.

OPERATIVE COURSE: After general endotracheal anesthesia, the patient was placed in the supine position. The right anterior neck areas were then prepared and draped in the usual fashion. An incision, which was running anterior to the border of the sternocleidomastoid muscles, was made using a #10 blade. Hemostasis was achieved using Bovie, which was used to transverse the platysma. Self-retaining retractors were placed. The plane anterior to the sternocleidomastoid muscle was then developed, using sharp and blunt dissection. Careful hemostasis was employed using bipolar cautery. The carotid sheath was then entered and the carotid and internal jugular veins were dissected out. The Henley retractor was placed. The carotid was dissected distally. There was no obvious common facial vein in the vicinity of the carotid bifurcation, which was, as predicted, highly placed. This necessitated careful and deliberate dissection distally, so as to preserve the hypoglossal nerve. This required division of the digastric muscle, using cautery. Great care was taken to identify and preserve the hypoglossal nerve. The need for careful preservation of this was attended to throughout the entire procedure. A small vein that was a tributary to the internal jugular vein was ligated and divided in this area as well.

A Rummel tourniquet was placed around the common carotid artery. 0 silk ties were placed around the internal and external carotid artery, and a 0 silk tie Potts ligature was placed around the first branch of the external carotid artery. There was no typically placed superior thyroid artery in this patient. It was unclear which branch of the external artery was thus represented as the first proximal branch that was identified. The carotid sinus nerves were infiltrated using 1% lidocaine in the area, and the bifurcation was extensively dissected out to allow for placement of these sutures around the vessels. A Hemovac drain was placed lateral to the carotid artery, and this was connected to suction. The patient was given 80 units/kg bolus of heparin. The internal, common, and external carotid arteries were test occluded, and there was no change in the EEG. The artery was then opened using a #11 blade. This was extended using Potts scissors. The plaque was shelled out in the usual fashion using #4 Penfield. The plaque was amputated proximally in the usual fashion by dividing it with a #11 blade after elevation using a right-angle clamp. The plaque was then removed from the external carotid artery using a standard eversion technique. The plaque was then dissected free at the internal carotid artery distally. An excellent break point was noted, and there did not appear to be any need for any intimal tack-up stitches placed.

The arteriotomy bed was then carefully inspected, and all flaky material was removed in standard fashion. The arteriotomy was then closed using running 6-0 Prolene suture. Prior to placement of the final sutures, internal/external carotid arteries were back-bled and heparinized saline was employed to remove any potential bubbles. The external and common were then unclamped, allowing perfusion out this route. The internal was subsequently unclamped, after it had been clamped for a total of 30 minutes. There was no change in the EEG or somatosensory of a potential monitoring during that time or at any other time during the operation. There appeared to be no worthy leakage from the

EXAM 4—SCENARIO 3 (*continued*)

arteriotomy site. The arteries were then inspected at great length with a Doppler to ensure an adequate signal. Thus, satisfied, we proceeded to close. The Hemovac drain was left in place. Great care was taken to ensure excellent hemostasis. In light of this rather atypical amount of ooze present, a partial reversal of the heparin was given by the anesthesiologist. The platysma was then closed using interrupted 2-0 Vicryl sutures. The skin was closed using a running 4-0 Monocryl suture. Steri-Strips and a dressing were applied. The patient was then extubated and taken to the recovery room in stable condition, moving all four extremities well.

Enter one diagnosis code and one procedure code.

DX1

PR1

EXAM 4—SCENARIO 4

DATE OF OPERATION: 11/01/20XX

PREOPERATIVE DIAGNOSIS: Left orbital pseudotumor

POSTOPERATIVE DIAGNOSIS: Left orbital pseudotumor

OPERATION: Anterior orbitotomy with a biopsy of lacrimal gland, left orbit

ANESTHESIA: General

SURGICAL INDICATIONS: The patient is a 10-year-old boy with a 2-year history of chronic inflammation of the left orbit including swelling of the medial and lateral recti muscles and the ipsilateral lacrimal gland and Tenon's capsule. Previous diagnostic studies included a normal CBC, C-reactive protein (less than 0.1), and C-ANCA and P-ANCA, which were negative suggesting there was no underlying vasculitis. Because of continued chronic inflammation for which he will probably need oral steroids, pretreatment biopsy of involved tissue was recommended. Brief review of the CT scan revealed that there was considerable enlargement of the lacrimal gland in the left orbit, therefore, biopsy of this tissue was recommended.

SURGICAL PROCEDURE: The child was brought to the operating room after adequate preoperative medications. He was induced with face mask anesthesia at which time an intravenous line was inserted, cardiac monitor, blood pressure cuff, EKG leads, and pulse oximeter were attached. The child was then intubated and maintained with an appropriate combination and mixture of anesthetic gases and oxygen compatible with general surgery. His face was prepared and draped in the usual sterile fashion.

Inspection of the left eyelid revealed that there was no crease. There was proptosis of the ipsilateral globe with fullness of the left upper eyelid. There seemed to be a previous scar in the left upper eyelid. Therefore the decision was made to position the anterior orbitotomy on the previous left upper eyelid scar. Therefore approximately a 2-cm area was demarcated with a marking pen in the superotemporal aspect of the upper eyelid above the area where the eyelid crease would normally be. The subcutaneous tissue was infiltrated with 1% Xylocaine with epinephrine. A #67 Beaver blade was used to incise the eyelid skin and superficial orbicularis. Prior to doing this, the eyelid was put on stretch by putting a 6-0 silk through the lash line and pulling the upper eyelid taut. Then the eyelid skin was tented up with small muscle hooks. The orbicularis muscle was incised centrally and then the incision in the orbicularis was extended to the medial and lateral margins of the skin incision. Hemostasis was obtained with bipolar cautery. The sharp dissection was continued posteriorly to the level of the orbital septum. The area of the orbital septum just at its junction with the lateral orbital rim was exposed using Ragnell retractors. The orbital septum was then incised and retracted. One could immediately see the orbital portion of the lacrimal gland prolapsed through the wound. The pseudocapsule of the lacrimal gland was separated on the posterior aspect of the gland. A small amount of tissue was tented up on forceps and excised using the #67 Beaver blade. The tissue was immediately sent to the histopathology laboratory as a fresh specimen for appropriate histopathology and immunohistochemistry as indicated. Hemostasis was obtained with digital pressure and topical application of Avitene.

Once hemostasis was obtained, the wound was closed in a two-layered approach. First a deep subcutaneous and orbicularis muscle was closed with 5-0 Vicryl, and then the skin was closed with several interrupted 6-0 plain. Topical ointment was placed on the wound. The child was then weaned from general anesthesia, extubated, and brought to the recovery room in good health without complications.

EXAM 4—SCENARIO 4 *(continued)*

PATHOLOGY REPORT

CLINICAL INFORMATION

PROCEDURE: Biopsy left orbital lesion

PREOPERATIVE DIAGNOSIS: Left orbital lesion

CLINICAL HISTORY: 10-year-old boy with chronic orbital inflammation (eye muscles, lacrimal gland) for 2 years

GROSS DESCRIPTION:

Received fresh designated LEFT LACRIMAL GLAND is a single, unoriented, irregular tan-pink portion of soft tissue measuring 0.8 × 0.6 × 0.1 cm, which is submitted entirely, intact, in one cassette.

MICROSCOPIC DESCRIPTION:

H&E-stained sections reveal a portion of lacrimal tissue, with well-organized lobules of glands separated by fibromuscular tissue bands. Occasional ducts are seen within the fibromuscular tissue. Scattered collections of lymphocytes, plasma cells, and eosinophils are present between the exocrine glands and in foci within the intervening fibrous bands. There is no evidence of a neoplastic process.

DIAGNOSIS: LEFT LACRIMAL GLAND, BIOPSY; LACRIMAL GLAND TISSUE WITH AT MOST MILDLY INCREASED INTERSTITIAL LYMPHOCYTES AND PLASMA CELLS (SEE COMMENT)

COMMENT: Normal lacrimal gland tissue contains scattered interstitial lymphocytes and plasma cells. The number of lymphocytes and plasma cells present in this biopsy are, at most, mildly increased. An infiltrative or neoplastic cell population is not identified.

Enter one diagnosis code and one procedure code.

DX1

PR1

EXAM 4—SCENARIO 5

INFUSION

DATE: 3/4/XX

LENGTH OF SERVICE: One and one-half hours

LOCATION: Emergency room

NOTES: A 45-year-old female patient presents to the emergency room with a diagnosed case of acute, severe gastroenteritis. She has been suffering for several days and presents today very dehydrated. Intravenous fluids have been ordered.

Enter two diagnosis codes and two procedure codes.

DX1

DX2

PR1

EXAM 4—SCENARIO 6

IMMUNIZATION

DATE: 2/25/XX

LOCATION: Physician's office

NOTES: A five-year-old child is seen in the physician's office to receive a DTaP immunization. A nurse reviews the child's immunization record with the mother then proceeds to check the child's temperature and other vital signs before proceeding to administer the immunization.

Enter one diagnosis and four procedure codes.

DX1

PR1

PR2

PR3

PR4

EXAM 4 – SCENARIO 7

REASON FOR VISIT: Patient comes in today for monitoring of his chronic obstructive pulmonary disease, but he is apparently having a flare-up that he thinks just started within the last day or so. There has been no fever or chills. He has had cough, but the sputum has been fairly clear. There is no chest pain, but it does feel tight. He has been more dyspneic, particularly with attempts to come to the office today. He's not had any trouble with edema. Patient has long-standing CLL.

MEDICATIONS:

1. Oxygen, 3 L/minute via nasal cannula continuously

2. Advair, 250/50, one inhalation q 12 h

3. Combivent, 2 puffs four times daily and as needed

4. Zyrtec, 10 mg daily, as needed

5. Prednisone, 5 mg daily

6. Norvasc, 10 mg daily

7. Tylenol No. 3 as needed

PHYSICAL EXAMINATION:

GENERAL: Pleasant, slightly cushingoid, elderly, white male in no distress, but he is definitely more tachypneic and labored with his speech than usual.

WEIGHT: 128

BLOOD PRESSURE: 170/80.

PULSE: 88 and regular

RESPIRATIONS: 16 to 18

NOSE: Nasal mucosa and turbinates clear

MOUTH: Clear

PHARYNX: Clear

NECK: Supple. No cervical or supraclavicular adenopathy.

LUNGS: Bilateral wheezes with poor air movement and prolonged expiratory phase; air movement is not as good as usual.

CARDIAC: Normal S1 and S2; I don't detect an S3

ABDOMEN: No tenderness

EXTREMITIES: No cyanosis, clubbing, or edema

LABORATORY: Oxygen saturation at rest on 3 L of oxygen with a conserver device is 96%. CBC today from laboratory is WNL.

EXAM 4—SCENARIO 7 (*continued*)

ASSESSMENT/PLAN:

1. COPD/chronic bronchitis, now with acute exacerbation. Treat with prednisone, 40 mg daily for 3 days then taper by 10 mg every third day; also treat empirically with Levaquin, 750 mg daily for 5 days.

2. Questionable asbestosis based on chest radiographic abnormalities, currently receiving disability compensation.

3. Chronic lymphocytic B-cell leukemia; in remission, will monitor again at next visit.

4. Anxiety disorder.

HISTORY: Detailed

EXAMINATION: Detailed

MEDICAL DECISION-MAKING: Moderate

Enter two diagnosis codes and one procedure code.

DX1

DX2

PR1

EXAM 4 – SCENARIO 8

SERVICE: Abdominal transplant

PREOPERATIVE DIAGNOSES: Persistent rejection and failed renal allograft with allograft nephropathy resulting in end-stage renal disease

POSTOPERATIVE DIAGNOSES: Persistent rejection and failed renal allograft with allograft nephropathy resulting in end-stage renal disease

OPERATIONS AND PROCEDURES: Transplant nephrectomy

ANESTHESIA: General endotracheal

INDICATIONS FOR THE OPERATION: The patient is a 25-year-old female who underwent a kidney transplant that subsequently failed due to persistent rejection. She has met end-stage criteria and is now being dialyzed. However, she continues to suffer persistent rejection despite triple immunosuppression. For this reason, she presents to the OR for elective-nephrectomy to take care of the above issues and also get her off of immunosuppression.

PROCEDURE: The patient was identified and brought to the operating room, placed in the supine position, and administered general endotracheal anesthetic. Her abdomen was shaved, prepared, and draped in a sterile fashion. She was explored through her previous right hockey stick incision. This was carried through the layers of the abdominal wall with care to avoid entrance into the peritoneal cavity. The kidney transplant was identified. The capsule was separated freeing the kidney circumferentially down to its vascular pedicle. Large vascular clamps were placed both from a superior and inferior position and crossclamped. The femoral artery pulse was checked and found to be 2+. The kidney was then amputated off its vascular pedicle above the clamps, and vessels were secured with two rows of running 3-0 Prolene. Cross-clamps were removed, and hemostasis was noted with no significant blood loss. The femoral artery was checked again, and it still had a 2+ pulse. Sutures were secured. Hemostasis was noted. The retroperitoneum was irrigated. Again, hemostasis was noted. A JP drain was placed subfascially through a right lower quadrant stab incision and secured to the skin with 2-0 nylon. The fascia was then closed in one layer using looped #1 PDS. The subcutaneous tissue was closed with 3-0 Vicryl, and the skin was closed with staples. A sterile dressing was applied, and the patient was extubated and transported to the recovery room in stable condition, having tolerated the procedure well.

ESTIMATED BLOOD LOSS: Less than 100 cc

Needle, sponge, and instrument counts correct.

SPECIMENS: Transplanted kidney

The patient received 250 cc of 5% albumin and 100 cc of normal saline.

Enter three diagnosis codes and one procedure code.

DX1

DX2

DX3

PR1

ANSWER KEY

Introductory Medical Scenarios

Scenario 1

DX1	Q30.8	Other congenital malformation of nose
PR1	15260	Full thickness graft, free, including direct closure of donor site, nose, ears, eyelids, and/or lips; 20 sq cm or less
PR2	21235	Graft; ear cartilage, autogenous, to nose or ear (includes obtaining graft)

Scenario 2

DX1	M24.151	Other articular cartilage disorders, right hip
PR1	29862	Arthroscopy, hip, surgical; with debridement/shaving of articular cartilage (chondroplasty), abrasion arthroplasty, and/or resection of labrum

Scenario 3

DX1	R10.84	Generalized abdominal pain
PR1	45380	Colonoscopy, flexible with biopsy, single or multiple
PR2	43239	Esophagogastroduodenoscopy, flexible, transoral; with biopsy, single or multiple

Scenario 4

DX1	J96.00	Acute respiratory failure, unspecified whether with hypoxia or hypercapnia
DX2	I62.9	Nontraumatic intracranial hemorrhage, unspecified
PR1	31600	Tracheostomy, planned (separate procedure)

Scenario 5

DX1	C50.911	Malignant neoplasm of unspecified site of right female breast
DX2	Z92.21	Personal history of antineoplastic chemotherapy
PR1	19307	Mastectomy, modified radical, including axillary lymph nodes, with or without pectoralis minor muscle, but excluding pectoralis major muscle

Scenario 6

DX1	J96.00	Acute respiratory failure, unspecified whether with hypoxia or hypercapnia
DX2	S27.329A	Contusion of lung, unspecified, initial encounter
DX3	B96.3	Haemophilus influenzae [H. influenzae] as the cause of diseases classified elsewhere
DX4	B37.1	Pulmonary candidiasis
PR1	99291	Critical care, evaluation and management of the critically ill or critically injured patient; first 30–74 minutes

Scenario 7

DX1	E06.3	Autoimmune thyroiditis
PR1	60220	Total thyroid lobectomy, unilateral; with or without isthmusectomy

Scenario 8

DX1	N18.6	End stage renal disease
DX2	Z99.2	Dependence on renal dialysis
PR1	36818	Arteriovenous anastomosis, open; by upper arm cephalic vein transposition

Scenario 9

DX1	G40.901	Epilepsy, unspecified, not intractable, with status epilepticus
PR1	95816	Electroencephalogram (EEG); including recording awake and drowsy

Scenario 10

DX1	H49.12	Fourth [trochlear] nerve palsy, left eye
PR1	70553	Magnetic resonance (eg, proton) imaging, brain (including brain stem); without contrast material, followed by contrast material(s) and further sequences

Scenario 11

DX1	S61.212A	Laceration without foreign body of right middle finger without damage to nail, initial encounter
PR1	99213	Office or other outpatient visit for the evaluation and management of an established patient, which requires a medically appropriate history and/or examination and low level of medical decision making
PR2	12001	Simple repair of superficial wounds of scalp, neck, axillae, external genitalia, trunk and/or extremities (including hands and feet); 2.5 cm or less

Scenario 12

DX1	N39.0	Urinary tract infection, site not specified
DX2	F20.9	Schizophrenia, unspecified
PR1	99203	Office or other outpatient visit for the evaluation and management of a new patient, which requires a medically appropriate history and/or examination and straightforward medical decision making
PR2	81025	Urine pregnancy test, by visual color comparison methods
PR3	81001	Urinalysis, by dip stick or tablet reagent for bilirubin, glucose, hemoglobin, ketones, leukocytes, nitrite, pH, protein, specific gravity, urobilinogen, any number of these constituents; automated, with microscopy

Scenario 13

DX1	Q17.0	Accessory auricle
DX2	Q18.1	Preauricular sinus and cyst
PR1	11442	Excision, other benign lesion, including margins, except skin tag (unless listed elsewhere), face, ears, eyelids, nose, lips, mucous membrane; excised diameter 1.1 to 2 cm
PR2	11200	Removal of skin tags, multiple fibrocutaneous tags, any area; up to and including 15 lesions
PR3	12051	Repair, intermediate, wounds of face, ears, eyelids, nose, lips and/or mucous membranes; 2.5 cm or less

Scenario 14

DX1	R00.2	Palpitations
DX2	Z98.890	Other specified postprocedural states
DX3	Z87.74	Personal history of (corrected) congenital malformations of heart and circulatory system
PR1	93224	External electrocardiographic recording up to 48 hours by continuous rhythm recording and storage; includes recording, scanning analysis with report, review and interpretation by a physician or other qualified health care professional

Scenario 15

DX1	O21.1	Hyperemesis gravidarum with metabolic disturbance
PR1	80048	Basic metabolic panel (Calcium, total)
PR2	85025	Blood count; complete (CBC), automated (Hgb, Hct, RBC, WBC and platelet count) and automated differential WBC count
PR3	36415	Collection of venous blood by venipuncture

Scenario 16

DX1	G45.9	Transient cerebral ischemic attack, unspecified
DX2	I34.1	Nonrheumatic mitral (valve) prolapse
PR1	99285	Emergency department visit for the evaluation and management of a patient, which requires these 3 key components within the constraints imposed by the urgency of the patient's clinical condition and/or mental status: a comprehensive history; a comprehensive examination; and medical decision making of high complexity
PR2	93010	Electrocardiogram, routine ECG with at least 12 leads; interpretation and report only

Scenario 17

DX1	S42.422A	Displaced comminuted supracondylar fracture without intercondylar fracture of left humerus, initial encounter for closed fracture
DX2	M08.20	Juvenile rheumatoid arthritis with systemic onset, unspecified site
PR1	99203	Office or other outpatient visit for the evaluation and management of a new patient, which requires a medically appropriate history and/or examination and low level of medical decision making
PR2	20670	Removal of implant; superficial (eg, buried wire, pin or rod) (separate procedure)

Scenario 18

DX1	K13.79	Other lesions of oral mucosa
PR1	40812	Excision of lesion of mucosa and submucosa, vestibule of mouth; with simple repair

Scenario 19

DX1	C79.51	Secondary malignant neoplasm of bone
DX2	C64.9	Malignant neoplasm of unspecified kidney, except renal pelvis
DX3	M84.552A	Pathological fracture in neoplastic disease, left femur, initial encounter for fracture
PR1	27236	Open treatment of femoral fracture, proximal end, neck, internal fixation or prosthetic replacement
PR2	27495	Prophylactic treatment (nailing, pinning, plating, or wiring) with or without methylmethacrylate, femur
PR3	27360	Partial excision (craterization, saucerization, or diaphysectomy) bone, femur, proximal tibia and/or fibula (eg, osteomyelitis or bone abscess)

Scenario 20

DX1	H71.91	Unspecified cholesteatoma, right ear
PR1	69643	Tympanoplasty with mastoidectomy (including canalplasty, middle ear surgery, tympanic membrane repair); with intact or reconstructed wall, without ossicular chain reconstruction

Exam 1

1. d   If the type of diabetes mellitus is not documented in the health record, the default is type 2 diabetes mellitus. The coding professional would also want to code the insulin use in addition to the diabetic code selected (Hazelwood and Venable 2014, 46; *ICD-10-CM Official Guidelines for Coding and Reporting 2022*, 1.C.4.a.2).

2. b   A radiologist's findings may be used to clarify an outpatient's diagnosis or reason for services. Based on the fact that the radiologist is a physician, a coding professional can use a diagnosis from the x-ray (*ICD-10-CM Official Guidelines for Coding and Reporting 2022*, IV.K).

3. b   Infants born to RH-negative mothers often develop hemolytic disease owing to fetal-maternal blood group incompatibility. These conditions are classified to Category P55, Hemolytic disease of newborn (Optum360 2022, 8; *ICD-10-CM Expert for Hospitals*, Alphabetic Index, main term Disease, subterm hemolytic).

4. a   When a patient has bilateral glaucoma and both eyes are documented as being the same type and stage, and the classification does not provide a code for bilateral glaucoma (namely, subcategories H40.10, and H40.20) report only one code for the type of glaucoma with the seventh character specifying the stage (*ICD-10-CM Official Guidelines for Coding and Reporting 2022*, I.C.7.a.2).

5. a   D53.9, K29.70—The signs and symptoms would not be coded as they are integral to the diagnoses of anemia and gastritis (*ICD-10-CM Official Guidelines for Coding and Reporting 2022*, 1.C.18.b).

6. b   E09.9, J84.9, K92.1, R09.02, M06.9, N18.9, T38.0X5A—DM caused by drug use is coded to category E09 (Leon-Chisen 2022, 163–164).

7. d   The patient experienced an adverse effect (drowsiness) due to sensitivity to the Periactin medication. The Adverse Effect column is selected from the Table of Drugs and Chemicals as the medication was taken as prescribed (Leon-Chisen 2022, 532–533).

8. a   In ICD-10-CM, the coding guideline for the sequelae or late effects is to code the residual condition (monoplegia) of the sequela first, followed by the cause of the sequela (poliomyelitis). Per the Coding Guidelines, when a scenario specifies monoplegia of an upper limb and does not identify whether the limb is the dominant or nondominant side, the default code for the affected left side is nondominant (*ICD-10-CM Official Guidelines for Coding and Reporting 2022*, I.B.10 and I.C.6.a).

9. b   During pregnancy, childbirth, or the puerperium, a patient admitted with a diagnosis of asymptomatic AIDS should receive a principal diagnosis of O98.72 and B20. (Once an individual has confirmed AIDS, code B20 must always be used in future hospital visits.) Code Z37.0 is for the live birth and Z3A.36 is for the specified (36) weeks of gestation (*ICD-10-CM Official Guidelines for Coding and Reporting 2022*, I.C.15.f).

10. c   A poisoning code (for the crack cocaine) is always sequenced first per the ICD-10-CM Coding Guidelines. In all of the other examples, the Acute Respiratory Failure is principal (*ICD-10-CM Official Guidelines for Coding and Reporting 2022*, 1.C.10.b.1; 1.C.19.e.5.b).

11. d   When a patient is diagnosed with an infection (such as pneumonia) that is due to MRSA, and that infection has a combination code that includes the causal agent, the appropriate combination code for that infection and its causal organism is assigned. If a patient has a current infection and a MRSA colonization, Z22.322 should also be assigned (*ICD-10-CM Official Guidelines for Coding and Reporting 2022*, 1.C.1.e.1).

12. a   When a patient is admitted for the purpose of having chemotherapy and develops a complication, such as nausea and vomiting, the principal diagnosis is still the admission for the chemotherapy (*ICD-10-CM Official Guidelines for Coding and Reporting 2022*, 1.C.2.e.3).

13. c   T81.42XA, B96.20, S82.201E—In this case, there is a wound infection following a surgical procedure. There is note under code T81.4XXA to use additional code to identify the infection and the organism identified was *E. coli,* which was coded as B96.20. The seventh character E was added to the fracture code to indicate routine fracture healing (Optum360 2022, *ICD-10-CM Expert for Hospitals* Tabular Index 2022, 1152).

14. c   In some cases symptoms are coded as additional diagnoses when they "represent important problems in medical care." With this question, it would be important to code the coma since it impacts the metastasis to the brain (Hazelwood and Venable 2014, 4; Schraffenberger and Palkie 2022, 38–39; *ICD-10-CM Official Guidelines for Coding and Reporting 2022* 1.C.18.e and 1.B.6).

15. a   To completely describe a pressure ulcer, use as many codes as needed from category L89 to identify the site of the pressure ulcer as well as the stage of the ulcer (*ICD-10-CM Official Guidelines for Coding and Reporting 2022*, I.C.12.a.1).

16. a   The Z38.00 code should be used because it was clearly stated that the baby was born vaginally. The fetal alcohol syndrome code should be used instead of the alcohol abuse code because the use of alcohol by the mother was manifested in the infant (Hazelwood and Venable 2014, 158).

17. c   The melanoma is coded to the site of the lesion (Alphabetic Index main term Melanoma, subterm Skin, subterm arm refers the coding professional to code C43.6–; C43.61 refers to malignant melanoma of right upper limb including shoulder) and the procedure code is determined based on the size of the lesion as well as the margins (Optum360 2022, *ICD-10-CM Expert for Hospitals*, Alphabetic Index, main term Melanoma; *CPT Assistant* Fall 1995, 3; May 1996, 11; Nov. 2002, 5; Feb. 2010, 3).

18. a   The coding notes before code 64490 state that bilateral injections should be coded using modifier 50. L2–L3 is the second lumbar level injected; therefore, 64494 is used in combination with 64493 (*CPT Professional Edition 2022*, 487).

19. c   The aortopulmonary septal defect, also called a fenestration (or hole), is an anomalous connection between the ascending aorta and the main pulmonary artery above the semilunar valves (the aortic and pulmonary valves). To eliminate the connection, the vessels are disconnected and a patch is placed to close the hole. In this case, the procedure is performed using a cardiopulmonary bypass machine, which diverts blood from the right side of the heart, through an oxygenating machine, and returns it to the left side of the circulation (*Mosby's* 2017, 122, 297).

20. c   Tests that are ordered together and performed together that are listed together as a panel must be billed as a panel. If all the tests listed in a panel are not performed, they must be billed individually. In this case, all of the tests listed in the electrolyte panel were performed and must be coded together as 80051 (Huey 2021, 246).

21. c   Code 22869 describes the work of placing the interspinous process distraction device without decompression or fusion (Huey 2021, 102–103).

22. c   The final closure is coded with 49606, after the repair of the gastroschisis is performed by placing a prosthesis over the protruding intestines (*CPT Assistant*, Winter 1994, 04(4): 12–17).

23. d   There are currently no codes that describe a CABG using a thoracoscopic approach, therefore the unlisted code is assigned (*CPT Professional Edition 2022*, 282).

24. c   Code 58262 describes the removal of a uterus 250 g or less, along with either one or both of the tubes and the ovaries (*CPT Professional Edition 2022*, 445).

25. b   This procedure is correctly described as code 31290 (*CPT Assistant*, Winter 1993, 04(3): 22–25).

26. d   Destruction codes are used because the physician curettes the lesions, which is included as a method of destruction. In addition, the lesions are actinic keratoses, which are listed as a form of premalignant lesions that are normally destroyed using this method (Huey 2021, 88).

27. b   This service requires a 99283 Emergency Department code (due to expanded problem-focused history), the code for the rabies immune globulin, and the administration and rabies vaccine and the vaccine administration (Huey 2021, 264–266, 319).

28. c   Reporting an office visit code is inappropriate if, during the course of events within a specific encounter, the physician admits the patient to the hospital (Huey 2021, 328).

29. b   The subcategories of preventive medicine services distinguish between new and established patients, with the individual codes identifying specified age ranges (Huey 2021, 346).

30. a   The facility will report only total time (85 minutes) using the codes for critical care (*CPT Assistant*, August 2016, 26(8): 9).

31. d   The correct code is 99213. The question states that the patient is an established patient, so codes should be chosen from the 99211–99215 range. According to the E/M coding changes implemented in January of 2021, the E/M level for office outpatients is based on either time or the revised level of medical decision-making. Here the physician documented 5 minutes reviewing the record from the primary physician, 15 minutes face-to-face with the patient, and 5 minutes documenting in the EHR. According to the guidelines, time does not have to be spent face-to-face with the patient. Therefore, the 5 minutes spent reviewing records and documenting in the EHR would be added to the 15 minutes spent face-to-face with the patient, for a total of 25 minutes. Code 99213 requires 20 to 29 minutes of total time spent on the date of the encounter (Huey 2021, 338–341).

32. c   It is appropriate to use an E/M code with modifier 57 when the physician determines during the E/M encounter that surgery is necessary (*CPT Assistant*, March 2015, 25(3): 3).

33. c   The sacral pressure ulcer is excised in preparation for two myocutaneous flaps, transferred from the buttocks on each side. Code 15936 describes the excision, and the myocutaneous flaps are not free grafts, but transfer flaps, coded as 15734 and 15734–59 (*CPT Assistant*, November 1998, 11(8): 6–7).

34. d   96413, 96417, 96367, J2405, J9045, J9267 × 25—This is an IV chemotherapy administration for greater than 30 minutes, which qualifies as up to one hour. The second infusion is also chemotherapy, for an additional hour as a sequential infusion. The third infusion is not chemotherapy and is coded as sequential infusion of a new drug. Code J2405 is coded as only one unit because the dose did not exceed the infused amount over the amount listed in the code description. Code J9267 is coded with a quantity of 25 units because the code description reads 1 mg (Huey 2021, 285–286).

35. c   Shoulder blade is a synonym of scapula; saucerization means excavation of tissue to form a shallow depression. This returns the shoulder blade to the natural contour as described in this case (*CPT Professional Edition 2022*, 172; *Mosby's* 2017, 459, 1621).

36. c   The only correct answer of these four is c, stating that you code all the laceration repairs (by adding together the lengths of those of the same site and complexity) and listing the code for the most complex repair first (Huey 2021, 82–83).

37. c   The left anterior descending artery and left circumflex are both considered "main" arteries, therefore, only base codes should be used. Codes must be sequenced according to the hierarchy provided in the CPT manual: 92943 = 92941 = 92933 > 92924 > 92937 = 92928 > 92920 (Huey 2021, 275–277; *CPT Professional Edition 2022*, 749–752).

38. b   The allergist provides single-dose vials as indicated in CPT code 95144 (Huey 2021, 280–281).

39. a   The coding professional chose the incorrect medication. Depo-Provera is used for estrogen replacement. The testosterone cypionate is a different medication (PDR 2021).

40. c   The only necessary information listed in the options is the reason for the thyroidectomy. CPT provides codes that describe thyroidectomy for malignancy and those without a stated reason (*CPT Professional Edition 2022*, 454).

41. c   According to the guidelines, in this situation, both codes may be payable if it is clinically appropriate and a PTP-associated modifier is used (CMS 2021b).

42. c   According to the National Correct Coding Initiative (NCCI), if a lesion is drained as part of another procedure, the incision and drainage is not separately reportable (CMS 2021b).

43. c   Although a layered closure may indicate the repair should be classified as intermediate, the extensive undermining increases the complexity of the procedure, meeting the definition of a complex repair (*CPT Professional Edition 2022*, 106–107).

44. c   Code 14020 includes excision of the benign lesion. The excision code (11402) should not be reported separately (*CPT Professional Edition 2022*, 109).

45. c   A surgical endoscopy includes a diagnostic endoscopy, so 43235 is not separately reportable. Because the physician dilated the esophagus with a balloon during endoscopy, 43249 most accurately describes the procedure (*CPT Professional Edition 2022*, 354–363).

46. d   Free skin grafts are coded based on the size and location of the defect at the recipient site. Simple repair of the donor site is not separately reportable (Huey 2021, 84–86).

47. a   There is no documentation to suggest this is a recurrent inguinal hernia repair. Do not code implantation of mesh separately with an inguinal hernia repair. Implantation of mesh can only be coded separately with an incisional or ventral hernia repair (*CPT Professional Edition 2022*, 400–401).

48. d   The therapeutic wedge resection was performed during thoracoscopy, therefore 32666 most accurately describes the procedure. Two of the other codes involve an open approach (thoracotomy) (Huey 2021, 114–115).

49. d   The procedure described is a uterus allotransplantation. Code 0667T includes transplantation of the uterus allograft and care of the recipient (*CPT Professional Edition 2022*, 912).

50. c   Each unit of the drug is worth 250 mg. 600 mg is more than 2 units and less than 3 units. Therefore, 3 units are reported (Huey 2021, 304).

51. c   The definition of "new patient" in CPT states that a new patient has not seen a physician from the exact same specialty and subspecialty within the same group practice within the past three years. Also, this patient is covered by Medicare and, therefore, consultation codes are not an option for coding purposes (Huey 2021, 312).

52. b   Hypothyroidism is a condition in which the thyroid gland does not make enough thyroid hormone. Levothyroxine (Synthroid) is commonly used to treat this condition (PDR 2022a).

53. c   Pathology reports are required for cases in which a surgical specimen is removed or expelled during a procedure. Specimens are examined both microscopically and macroscopically (Reynolds and Morey 2020, 115).

54. d   According to CMS, all of the above may provide CCM services using CPT code 99490 (*CPT Professional Edition 2022*, 64–65).

55. d.   While published by the American Hospital Association, the Coding Handbook is not considered an authoritative source by CMS (Casto and White 2021, 182).

56. b   As clinical documentation improvement staff review documentation, situations where a query may be necessary include when documentation provides a diagnosis without supporting clinical validation (Hunt and Kirk 2020, 287).

57. c   The coding professional should not indicate to the physician that a different diagnosis, not supported by the health record, would increase reimbursement (Handlon 2020, 287).

58. b   Documentation that is clear thoroughly describes what is occurring with the patient. Consistent documentation does not contradict itself. Documentation that is reliable is trustworthy. Complete documentation is detailed and has maximum content fully addressing all concerns in the record (Handlon 2020, 287).

59. c   CPT code 45388, Colonoscopy, flexible; with ablation of tumor(s), polyp(s), or other lesion(s) (include pre- and post-dilation and guide wire passage, when performed), is used when a neodymium yttrium aluminum garnet (Nd:YAG) laser is used (Huey 2021, 146).

60. b   Excision of a skin lesion includes simple repair, so simple repair should not be coded separately. However, when a layered or intermediate repair is performed following removal of a skin lesion, the intermediate repair code should be reported in addition to the excision code. Adjacent tissue transfer includes excision of a lesion (Huey 2021, 80–81, 84).

61. b   Wound debridement codes are selected based on the depth of tissue removed, and the surface area of the wound (*CPT Professional Edition 2022*, 95).

62. d   Coding policies should include the following components: AHIMA Code of Ethics, AHIMA Standards of Ethical Coding, Official Coding Guidelines, applicable federal and state regulations, and internal documentation policies requiring the presence of physician documentation to support all coded diagnosis and procedure code assignments (Hunt and Kirk 2020, 297).

63. d   Assign a code for the chief complaint as the reason for the visit in the absence of a diagnosis or defined problem, the chief compliant should be coded as the reason for the visit (*ICD-10-CM Official Guidelines for Coding and Reporting 2022*, IV.D).

64. b   HIPAA provides for criminal penalties for healthcare professional who "knowingly and willingly" attempt to defraud any health program (Huey 2021, 430–431).

65. a   For symptomatic individuals with actual or suspected exposure to COVID-19 and the infection has been ruled out, assign code Z20.822 for contact with and (suspected) exposure to COVID-19. Instruction under J18 reminds the coding professional to code both the pneumonia and the influenza (*ICD-10-CM Official Guidelines for Coding and Reporting 2022,* I.C.g.1.e; I.C.21.c.1).

66. c   For a patient with pneumonia confirmed as due to COVID-19, assign U07.1 and J12.89. For the sepsis, the sepsis code is assigned as an additional code as it developed on day 3 (*ICD-10-CM Official Guidelines for Coding and Reporting 2022,* 1.C.1.g).

67. d   The coding trainee made two errors. First, squamous cell carcinoma indicates a malignant lesion. Therefore, an excision code from the malignant lesion range should have been used (11600–11646). Second, the trainee failed to add the margins properly to indicate the total size of the excised lesion (3.0 cm + 1.0 cm + 1.0 cm = 5.0 cm) (*CPT Professional Edition 2022*, 101–105).

68. c   There is clear documentation of an arthroscopy with limited debridement, so that procedure should be coded regardless of the operative statement. Documentation supports the surgical arthroscopy code. Also, surgical endoscopy always includes a diagnostic arthroscopy, therefore 29830 should not be reported separately (*CPT Professional Edition 2022*, 212–213).

69. c   This is an example of assessment; a is monitor, b is evaluate, and d is treatment (Watson 2018, 46).

70. b   The purpose of the HCC model is to predict future costs for patients with chronic conditions and ensure proper funding for government healthcare plans (Watson 2018, 46).

71. c   The HIPAA Privacy and Security Rules apply to PHI used or disclosed by covered entities. Covered entities are healthcare providers, healthcare clearinghouses, and health plans that conduct the financial and administrative transactions described in the Transaction and Code Sets Rule (TCS). If an individual provider or an organization does not fit within the definitions of a healthcare provider, clearinghouse, or health plan, the rules do not apply (Brinda and Watters 2020, 317).

72. a   The request may be denied if it is determined that the PHI or the record was accurate and complete as it stands (Rinehart-Thompson 2017b, 246–247).

73. d   Regardless of whether the patient is an adult or a minor, the law allows a presumption of consent during an emergency situation (Klaver 2017, 144).

74. d   The designated record set is a group of records maintained by a covered entity and used in whole or in part to make decisions about an individual. Individuals may obtain a copy of PHI in the designated record set (Rinehart-Thompson. 2017a, 217).

75. c   Modifier AI is required for patients covered by Medicare when reporting Initial Hospital Service codes and this modifier is missing from the code (Huey 2021, 328).

76. a   According to the CPT book, these codes are used when the cast or strapping is an initial service without restorative treatment (*CPT Professional Edition 2022*, 210).

77. d   The physician's own office is considered a nonfacility and the physician incurs the costs of personnel, supplies, and equipment (Casto and White 2021, 122–123).

78. c   This is considered a facility, so the correct formula is: $6.71 \times 1.032 + 2.55 \times 1.130 + .78 \times 607 = 10.2796 \times \$36.88 = \$379.11$ (Casto and White 2021, 122–124).

79. a   These types of services are considered "Incident to" and the physician will bill for the service and receive the full Medicare Fee Schedule amount (Casto and White 2021, 126).

80. c   Audiologists, midwives, and psychologists practicing within their scope of practice and within state laws may receive payment under RBRVS (Casto and White 2021, 124–125).

81. a   According to the Place of Service code set by cms.gov, an urgent care facility is considered a nonfacility.

82. b   Choice B is leading the physician to document sepsis in the record (ACDIS-AHIMA 2019).

83. a   Physician's bill using the CPT codes regardless of the place of service (Casto and White 2021, 122).

84. d   While manual review, coding professionals, and compliance auditors are all ways of identifying errors prior to claims submission, most facilities use various types of editing software such as scrubbers or NCCI edits to review claims prior to submission (Casto and White 2021, 167).

85. b   Adjudication is the determination of the reimbursement amount based on the beneficiary's insurance plan benefits. Four outcomes may occur from adjudication: payment, suspend, reject, or deny. A reject outcome can occur at the claim level or the line-item level. The payer may reject single or multiple line items on the claim but approve payment for the remaining lines (Casto and White 2021, 171).

86. a The Medicare Claims Processing Manual is one of many manuals included in the CMS Internet-Only Manuals System that is used by the CMS program components to administer CMS programs. The CMS Program transmittals are used by CMS to communicate policies and procedures for the various payment systems' program manuals to the MACs. National coverage determinations are rules that are released by CMS that describe the circumstances under which supplies, services, or procedures are covered nationwide while local coverage determinations are used to determine coverage within the jurisdiction of a MAC rather than nationwide. The NCCI is a set of edits that was designed to promote national correct coding practices and to control improper coding that results in inappropriate payment for Part B claims (Casto and White 2021, 214).

87. c Dr. Smith receives 80 percent of the Medicare allowed amount, which is $160. Dr. Jones receives nothing from CMS because he does not accept assignment. The patient receives the benefits (Huey 2021, 371).

88. c Dr. Smith will receive the entire $200 minus $160 from CMS and the remaining 20 percent or $40 from the patient. Dr. Jones will receive $218.50 from the patient. This amount is the most he can charge under CMS's limiting charge rule. This figure is derived by determining the non-PAR allowed charge, which is 95 percent of the PAR amount—in this case, that would be $190. The limiting charge = 115% of that amount or $218.50 (Huey 2021, 371).

89. a The insurer will send the patient an Explanation of Benefits, which describes how a payment on a claim was made. The Remittance Advice is sent to the provider and the Medicare Explanation of Benefits is now called the Medicare Summary Notice (Casto and White 2021 172–173).

90. a The insurer sends the Remittance Advice to the provider to indicate how payment was made on the claim. The Advance Beneficiary Notice is used to document that Medicare may not pay for a service. The Explanation of Benefits is sent to the patient (Casto and White 2021, 172).

91. d The conversion factor is an across-the-board multiplier that is determined each year. It transforms the total of the RVUs into a payment amount (Casto and White 2021, 123).

92. d The practice expense includes payroll, office expenses, medical materials and supplies, and such (Casto and White 2021, 122–123).

93. a Local Coverage Determinations of LCDs are coverage policies that designate which ICD-10-CM codes establish medical necessity for various HCPCS codes. MACs publish local or regional determinations while National Coverage Determinations or NCDs refer to all providers in the country (Handlon 2020, 247).

94. b Medicare coverage is limited to items and services that are considered to be medically necessary for the diagnosis or treatment of a patient's condition. Coverage policies refer to whether a service is covered by Medicare. Precertification refers to the process of predetermining coverage before a service is done (Handlon 2020, 248).

95. b An EGD is not advanced to the jejunum. Colonic polyps would be found on a colonoscopy and pharyngitis would not require an EGD to diagnose. However, an EGD would be used to diagnose and treat duodenal ulcers (*CPT Professional Edition 2022*, 354).

96. b   The clean claim rate assesses the ability to comply with billing edits. The denial rate is the measure that assesses the ability to comply with documentation, coding, and billing requirements. The PEPPER metric is used to identify billing patterns different from the majority of other providers in the nation. The capture rate is the metric used to identify coding of secondary diagnoses (Casto and White 2021, 197).

97. c   The physician response rate is how long it takes for a physician to respond to a CDI query. The physician clarification rate is the number of clarifications placed by a CDI intervention that had an impact on the code and the physician agreement with CDI specialist rate is the number of times a physician agrees with a CDI intervention divided by the number of CDI interventions issued (Casto and White 2021, 195).

CCS-P MEDICAL SCENARIOS

Exam 1 Scenario 1

DX1	E10.10	Type 1 diabetes mellitus with ketoacidosis without coma
DX2	J45.909	Unspecified asthma, uncomplicated
PR1	99476	Subsequent inpatient pediatric critical care, per day, for the evaluation and management of a critically ill infant or young child, 2 through 5 years of age

Exam 1 Scenario 2

DX1	J45.909	Unspecified asthma, uncomplicated
DX2	M94.0	Chondrocostal junction syndrome [Tietze]
DX3	K21.9	Gastro-esophageal reflux disease without esophagitis
DX4	G43.909	Migraine, unspecified, not intractable, without status migrainosus
PR1	99285	Emergency department visit for the evaluation and management of a patient, which requires these 3 key components within the constraints imposed by the urgency of the patient's clinical condition and/or mental status: a comprehensive history; a comprehensive examination; and medical decision making of high complexity

Exam 1 Scenario 3

DX1	M51.16	Intervertebral disc disorders with radiculopathy, lumbar region
DX2	G89.29	Other chronic pain
PR1	63650	Percutaneous implantation of neurostimulator electrode array, epidural

Exam 1 Scenario 4

DX1	C61	Malignant neoplasm of prostate
DX2	C77.2	Secondary and unspecified malignant neoplasm of intra-abdominal lymph nodes
PR1	54520	Orchiectomy, simple (including subcapsular), with or without testicular prosthesis, scrotal or inguinal approach

Exam 1 Scenario 5

DX1	F90.9	Attention-deficit hyperactivity disorder, unspecified type
DX2	F43.22	Adjustment disorder with anxiety
PR1	90837	Psychotherapy, 60 minutes with patient

Exam 1 Scenario 6

DX1	Z51.11	Encounter for antineoplastic chemotherapy
DX2	C19	Primary neoplasm of rectosigmoid junction
PR1	96413	Chemotherapy administration, intravenous infusion technique; up to 1 hour; single or initial substance/drug
PR2	96417	each additional sequential infusion (different substance/drug), up to 1 hour (List separately in addition to code for primary procedure)
PR3	96374	Therapeutic, prophylactic, or diagnostic injection (specify substance or drug); intravenous push, single or initial substance/drug

Exam 1 Scenario 7

DX1	D49.1	Neoplasm of unspecified behavior of respiratory system
PR1	31625	Bronchoscopy, rigid or flexible, including fluoroscopic guidance, when performed; with bronchial or endobronchial biopsy(s), single or multiple sites

Exam 1 Scenario 8

DX1	J18.9	Pneumonia, unspecified organism
PR1	99239	Hospital discharge day management; more than 30 minutes

Exam 2

1. d   In addition to code Z33.2 (Encounter for elective termination of pregnancy), a code for the outcome of delivery category Z37 may be assigned (*ICD-10-CM Official Guidelines for Coding and Reporting 2022*, 1.C.15.q.1).

2. c   Code P70.1, Syndrome of infant of a diabetic mother, should be assigned when the newborn infant of a diabetic mother manifests features of this condition (Leon-Chisen 2022, 169).

3. b   When a patient has bilateral glaucoma and each eye is documented as having a different type or stage and the classification distinguishes laterality, assign the appropriate code for each eye rather than the code for bilateral glaucoma (*ICD-10-CM Official Guidelines for Coding and Reporting 2022*, 1.C.7.a.3).

4. c   ICD-10-CM's Alphabetic Index lists Ulcer as the main term with the subterm decubitus. There is a note that refers the coding professional to *see* Ulcer, pressure, by site. Referring to main term Ulcer again with subterms pressure, sacral region lists the code as L89.159. Code L89.150 refers to an unstageable pressure ulcer of the sacral region (*ICD-10-CM Official Guidelines for Coding and Reporting 2022*, 1.C.12.a).

5. a   The urinary tract infection was diagnosed on a 20-year-old patient, not a newborn, and the urine culture indicated *Shiga* toxin-producing *E. coli* O157 so neither the "unspecified" nor the "other specified" *E. coli* codes would be appropriate. In the Alphabetic Index, refer to Escherichia coli, O157 to locate B96.21. To locate this code in the Alphabetic Index, look up the main term Infection with subterm urinary (tract) and the code is listed (N39.0). In the Tabular List, there is a note to use additional code to code the infectious agent (Hazelwood and Venable 2014, 19; Optum360 2022, *ICD-10-CM Expert for Hospitals*).

6. d   Z51.11, C56.9, C78.00, C79.31—Code Z51.11 would be the first-listed code to indicate that the reason for the encounter is chemotherapy. The codes indicating the neoplasm sites would also be reported. In the Alphabetic Index, reference the main term Carcinoma with subterms papillary, serous, unspecified site which references code C56.9. The secondary sites (lungs and brain) can be located in the Neoplasm Table (*ICD-10-CM Official Guidelines for Coding and Reporting 2021*, 1.C.2.e.2; Optum360 2022, *ICD-10-CM Expert for Hospitals*).

7. c   When a physician refers to "deep" burns he is referring to third degree burns that extend through the skin into the underlying fascia and may damage the tendons and bones (Leon-Chisen 2022, 525).

8. a   If a patient has received tPA within the 24 hours prior to admission, the claim submitted by the physician at the specialty hospital will include Z92.82. This is a physician claim rather than the coding professional at hospital #2. The condition requiring the tPA administration, in this case the MI (code I21.09), is coded first. Code I22.0 is not used because this refers to a subsequent infarction. Chest pain is a symptom of a myocardial infarction and would, thus, not be coded (*ICD-10-CM Official Guidelines for Coding and Reporting 2022*, 1.C.9.e).

9. b   Code only the acute myocardial infarction (code I21.09) at the first hospital encounter since this is when the patient was first diagnosed in the ED. Code I22.0 would not be used because this code refers to a subsequent infarction that the patient did not have in this particular case. Chest pain would not be coded because it is a symptom of an acute myocardial infarction and the infarction is coded instead (Leon-Chisen 2021, 403–405).

10. d   There is a specific code that should be assigned—R87.615, Unsatisfactory cytologic smear of cervix (Schraffenberger and Palkie 2022, 573).

11. c   Nonhealing burns are coded as acute burns (*ICD-10-CM Official Guidelines for Coding and Reporting 2022*, 1.C.19.d.3).

12. b   K80.00, R00.0, Z53.09—When a surgery is planned but canceled, the code for the condition is still coded first. In addition, the contraindication is also coded, as well as Z53.09, to indicate the canceled surgery (Schraffenberger and Palkie 2022, 701).

13. c   C61, N40.1, R33.8—In addition to coding the BPH with lower urinary tract symptoms (LUTS), code the adenocarcinoma and per the instructional guideline at N40.1, an additional code is assigned for the urinary retention (Optum360 2022, *ICD-10-CM Expert for Hospitals*, code N40.1).

14. b   The residual condition (namely, the perineum prolapsed) is to be sequenced first per instructional notes at O94 (Hazelwood and Venable 2014, 151; *ICD-10-CM Official Guidelines for Coding and Reporting 2022*, 1.C.15.p).

15. c   The postprocedural hypoinsulinemia (E89.1) is the first-listed code followed by the code E13.9, Other specified diabetes mellitus without complications, and finally code Z90.411 for acquired partial absence of pancreas (*ICD-10-CM Official Guidelines for Coding and Reporting 2022*, 1.C.4.a.6.b.i).

16. d   Code C44.211 is the correct code. The first step in coding neoplasms is to reference the Alphabetic Index under the main term. In this case, the main term Carcinoma is referenced followed by subterm basal cell. A cross reference note directs the coding professional to Skin, subterms ear, basal cell carcinoma. The Tabular List is consulted to complete the code (Hazelwood and Venable 2014, 31–32; *ICD-10-CM Official Guidelines for Coding and Reporting 2022*, 1.C.2).

17. b   Codes 86769 and 86238 are used for antibody testing. Code 87635 is used for infectious agent detection (*CPT Professional Edition* 2022, 683).

18. c   See Coding Guidelines codes 33202–33249 (*CPT Professional Edition 2022*, 248–250).

19. b   "All PCI procedures performed in all segments (proximal, mid, distal) of a single major coronary artery through the native coronary circulation are reported with one code." The blockage is not total, and there is no associated myocardial infarction documented (*CPT Professional Edition 2022*, 749–752).

20. c   Based on the documentation, the physician would use the level of medical decision-making to select the level of E/M code. The number and complexity of problems addressed would be moderate (one undiagnosed new problem with uncertain prognosis). The amount and or complexity of data to be reviewed and analyzed is minimal (only one test ordered). The risk of complications and/or morbidity or mortality of patient management is moderate (prescription drug management). Since two of the three elements of medical decision-making are at the moderate level, the overall level of medical decision-making is moderate, which is included in the description of code 99204 (Huey 2021, 338–341).

21. c　The documentation includes that the bone fragments pierced the dura; therefore, repair of the dura must be included in the code(s) assigned. Cranioplasty is not described in the documentation. Code 62010 for the elevation of the depressed skull fracture with repair of dura and/or debridement of brain describes the performed procedures, indexed under Fracture, skull (*CPT Professional Edition 2022*, 469).

22. d　The coding professional should always reference the codes found in the Tabular before code assignment (Huey 2021, 22).

23. a　Code 36901 describes the work of accessing and imaging the AV shunt. Ultrasound guidance is included in 36901 (*CPT Professional Edition 2022*, 317–319).

24. b　Hallux rigidus is arthritis of the metatarsophalangeal joint, which is resected and replaced with an implant, described by code 28291 (Huey 2021, 103–104; *CPT Professional Edition 2022*, 205–206).

25. a　64635, 64636—Injection of a destructive agent into a facet joint nerve is coded with the code series 64633–64636. The fluoroscopic guidance is not coded separately, based on a coding note found at 77003. Code series 64493–64495 and 0216T–0218T are not used for injection of destructive agents, and the Category III codes are not applicable because they require ultrasound guidance (*CPT Professional Edition 2022*, 491–492).

26. d　Preventive medicine services category codes are assigned based on the age of the patient (Huey 2021, 346).

27. b　The 2021 revisions to E/M coding guidelines that allow time to be used for code selection apply to visits in the office or other outpatient visit categories (99202–99205 and 99211–99215) (Huey 2021, 338–341).

28. b　This is the definition of the codes used to describe admission and discharge on the same calendar date (*CPT Professional Edition 2022*, 25).

29. c　Code 36589 should be used for removal of tunneled catheters only. Removal of a catheter not requiring a surgical procedure does not warrant assignment of a separate code. CPT code 99213 requires documentation of a medically appropriate history and physical exam, and low-level medical decision-making (Huey 2021, 132).

30. c　A combination code exists for observation or inpatient care services involving admit and discharge on the same day. These codes require all three key components be met. Due to the fact that the medical decision-making was of low complexity, code 99234 must be assigned (Huey 2021, 328–329).

31. b　This question is the classic description of two surgeons performing one procedure (Huey 2021, 58).

32. b　The only modifier in the list that is eligible for use with an E/M code is modifier 32 (Huey 2021, 322–323).

33. c　This question defines a domiciliary. It is used to report evaluation and management services in a facility that provides room, board, and other personal assistance services, generally on a long-term basis (*CPT Professional Edition 2022*, 36–38).

34. d   This injection is transforaminal. A coding note at 64484 states that these procedures are unilateral and modifier 50 should be appended to 64483 if the procedure is performed bilaterally. However, do not append modifier 50 to 64484. Instead, report the add-on code twice. The guidance used is fluoroscopy; therefore, the 64483 is assigned for the first level (L4) and 64484 is assigned for the additional level (L5) (*CPT Professional Edition 2022*, 484–487).

35. c   The patient is identified as a "longtime" patient, implying that the patient is established with this physician. Only time spent on the date of the encounter can be counted toward total time for office and other outpatient visit code selection (Huey 2021, 338–341).

36. b   The most complicated wound repair must be sequenced first, followed by the less complicated wound repair. Modifier 59 must be appended to secondary procedures. Modifier LT is should not be used with wound repair codes (*CPT Professional Edition 2022*, 106–109).

37. c   Implantation of mesh following an incisional or ventral hernia repair should be reported separately using the add-on code 49568. Add-on codes should never be sequenced first or used alone (Huey 2021, 153).

38. b   CPT describes x-rays based on the number of views, or positions in which the images are taken, not the actual number of images, or pictures, that were taken. The anteroposterior is one view and the lateral is another view. Therefore, code 71046 is assigned for two views (Huey 2021, 224).

39. b   One of the uses of the molecular pathology procedures is to test for histocompatibility antigens. The tests in this section are qualitative, not quantitative, and there are only two tiers of tests. The Bethesda system is used to report cytopathology results, not molecular pathology (*CPT Professional Edition 2022*, 616–619; *CPT Changes 2012: An Insider's View*, 147).

40. a   Per CPT Guidelines, if a diagnostic colonoscopy is attempted, but fails to reach the splenic flexure, it must be coded as a diagnostic sigmoidoscopy, 45330 (*CPT Professional Edition 2022*, 381).

41. b   When offenses are discovered, they should be investigated, and corrective measures undertaken. Physician practices should develop indicators that would signal a problem. Corrective action may include refunding overpayments from a third-party payer or even self-reporting to the government (Hazelwood and Venable 2014, 231–232).

42. b   According to the National Correct Coding Initiative (NCCI), when an arthroscopy is converted to an open procedure, only the open procedure may be reported (CMS 2021b).

43. c   To accurately assign a code for hernia repair, the coding professional must identify the type of hernia (umbilical), the age of the patient (three years old), the history of the hernia (initial), and the clinical presentation of the hernia (reducible) (Huey 2021, 151–152).

44. b   If, during cystoscopy, a temporary stent is inserted and removed, it should not be reported separately (Huey 2021, 162–163).

45. c   Destruction/excision of lesions of the penis are not coded from the integumentary section of CPT, but from the male genital section. There is no documentation to support the use of modifier 22 (Huey 2021, 169).

46. c   The coding professional must first determine if the vaginal hysterectomy is done via a laparoscope or open. Size of the uterus must also be noted. The salpingo-oophorectomy is included in the hysterectomy code and should not be reported separately (Huey 2021, 172–175).

47. d   Both codes 92924 and 92928 include a PTCA when performed, so codes 92920 and /92921 would not be reported separately. Since both vessels are considered major coronary arteries, base codes would be used. The add-on codes are used for branches (*CPT Professional Edition 2022*, 749–751).

48. c   The physician would report the procedure, appending a modifier 53 indicating the procedure was discontinued due to circumstances that threatened the well-being of the patient. Modifier 74 would not be used by a physician, but by the hospital or surgery center (*CPT Professional Edition 2022*, 918–922).

49. d   The codes are differentiated according to the route of administration. For Medicare cases, a Level II HCPCS code (J series) is reported with the identification of the specific substance or drug. In this case, use both 96372 and J0561 (Huey 2021, 304).

50. b   Medicare uses unique procedural codes to identify claims for services when colonoscopy is performed strictly for colorectal neoplasia screening in patients with average risk (G0121, Colorectal cancer screening; colonoscopy on individual not meeting criteria for high risk) and high risk (G0105, Colorectal cancer screening; colonoscopy on individual at high risk) for colon cancer. This patient has no history and is therefore not high risk. In these cases, G0121 is reported instead of the standard CPT diagnostic colonoscopy code when there is no need for a therapeutic procedure (*CPT Assistant*, January 2004, 07(14): 4–25).

51. c   The documentation as a result of the query should be included in the patient record to communicate to other providers and support the patient's course of treatment (Hunt and Kirk 2020, 289).

52. c   The total size of a removed lesion, including margins, is needed for accurate coding. This information is best provided in the operative report. The pathology report typically provides the specimen size rather than the size of the excised lesion. Because the specimen tends to shrink, this is not an accurate measurement (Huey 2021, 80–81).

53. d   The coding professional should reference the NCCI, as it is the authority on PTP edits to prevent inappropriate payment of services that should not be reported together (CMS 2021b).

54. a   The most accurate documentation of the total size of the excised area should be taken from the operative report. The pathology report will include specimen size, which may reflect some shrinkage. The anesthesia record and nurses notes would be unlikely to include total size of the excised lesion (Huey 2021, 80).

55. c   Per the Official Guidelines (Section IV.M), choice c is correct. For patients receiving diagnostic or therapeutic services, sequence first the diagnosis shown in the medical record to be chiefly responsible for the services provided. Uncertain diagnoses are not reported in the outpatient setting (*ICD-10-CM Official Guidelines for Coding and Reporting 2022*, IV.H, IV.K, IV.L, IV.M).

56. c   Haldol is used to treat symptoms of schizophrenia. More information on Haldol is available at Prescribers' Digital Reference (PDR 2022b).

57. a   Queries may be either verbal or written. Verbal queries may be made in person or over the telephone (Handlon 2020, 288).

58. a   This would be leading the physician to a diagnosis of sepsis (Handlon 2020, 290).

59. d   Status asthmaticus is an acute asthmatic attack in which the degree of bronchial obstruction is not relieved by usual treatments such as epinephrine or aminophylline. A patient in status asthmaticus fails to respond to therapy (Leon-Chisen 2022, 234–235). Only a physician can diagnose status asthmaticus. If a coding professional suspects the condition based on the symptoms documented in the health record, the coding professional should query the physician about the documentation for status asthmaticus.

60. a   Modifier 25 may be used to report a significant, separately identifiable evaluation and management service by the same physician on the day of a procedure or other service. Different diagnoses are not required for reporting the evaluation and management service (Huey 2021, 322–323).

61. d   In order to accurately code CVAD, the coding professional must determine: Was the catheter inserted centrally or peripherally? Was it tunneled or nontunneled? Was a port or pump used? What is the age of the patient? The other terms are associated with other cardiac procedures (Huey 2021, 132–133).

62. c   Developing, coordinating, and participating in coding training programs falls under the area of monitoring compliance efforts of the practice, whereas the other answers are actual risk areas identified by the OIG (Hazelwood and Venable 2014, 231–232).

63. c   Medicare defines "abuse" as involving billing practices that are inconsistent with generally acceptable fiscal policies. This usually results from inadvertent coding or billing mistakes and is not considered fraudulent (Hazelwood and Venable 2014, 231).

64. c   The OIG investigates and prosecutes individuals who overbill Medicare and also develops an annual "work plan" that lists specific "target areas" monitored in a given year (Huey 2021, 431–433).

65. a   During quantitative analysis, the record is reviewed for completeness and accuracy. It is most likely that missing signatures would be discovered during this type of review. While there may be some overlap between quantitative and qualitative analysis, qualitative analysis requires a more in-depth review for quality and adequacy of documentation (Reynolds and Morey 2020, 125–126).

66. c   Allowing the physician to select the codes for an audit will not ensure a representative sample (Huey 2021, 426–427).

67. d   Codes from the range 33510 to 33516 should not be used for combined arterial-venous grafts. Code 33534 must be reported first. Code 33518 is an add-on code, which should never be sequenced first (*CPT Professional Edition 2022*, 264–267).

68. b   Critical care less than 30 minutes should be reported with the appropriate E/M code. Emergency department codes require all three key components be met. Therefore, 99284 should be assigned (*CPT Professional Edition 2022*, 32–33).

69. c   The CMS-HCC model does not include acute illnesses and injuries that are not predictive of ongoing healthcare costs (Watson 2018, 49).

70. a   This is an example of appropriate treatment documentation; b is an assessment; c is an example of evaluate; and d is an example of assessment (Watson 2018, 46).

71. d   There are certain exceptions where the minimum necessary requirement does not apply and the individual or the individual's personal representation is one of the exceptions (Brinda and Watters 2020, 318).

72. a   The notice should be given at the initial contact (Reynolds and Morey 2020, 108).

73. d   Disclosure to a family member can be made only in accordance with a properly executed authorization form (Rinehart-Thompson 2017a, 221–230).

74. b   The Notice of Privacy Practices explains TPO uses and disclosures (Rinehart-Thompson 2017a, 219).

75. c   The only true statement listed there is the fact that surgical preparation codes can be used with graft, flap, or skin substitute codes. They are used for wounds to be healed by primary intention, are not the same as debridement codes, and can be used with wounds to be treated by negative-pressure wound therapy (*CPT Assistant* March 2008, 18(3): 14–15; Huey 2021, 85–86).

76. a   This production report does not contain any entries for new patient E/M codes. It is highly unlikely that all patients that have not been seen previously were seen at the request of another healthcare provider. Therefore, the physician may require education on the definition of new patient visits (Huey 2021, 409–413).

77. c   A is not correct as the RVU for a nonfacility is higher than for a facility; the selection for place of service is dependent on several factors; there are six categories of PE as identified by CMS (Casto and White 2021, 122–123).

78. a   The correct formula for a "facility" is $4.78 \times 1 + 3.75 \times .889 + .48 \times .707 = 8.453$ (Casto and White 2021, 122–123).

79. c   Because the physician is not on the premises, this cannot be considered incident to billing; therefore, the PA must bill under his own NPI and receive 85 percent of the MPFS amount (Casto and White 2021, 125–126).

80. a   In this situation considering that all "incident to" requirements are met, the claim can be submitted using the physician's NPI (Casto and White 2021, 125–126).

81. d   Single path coding is a process where one coding professional assigns the codes required for both facility and professional claims during the same coding session. It does eliminate duplicative processes and productivity is optimized. It also enhances coding accuracy (Casto and White 2021, 163).

82. c   Adjudication is the determination of the reimbursement amount based on the beneficiary's insurance plan benefits. Four outcomes may occur from adjudication: payment, suspend, reject, or deny. A denial outcome may be a claim denial or line-item denial. A denial indicates that the provider must go through the appeals process if he or she disagrees with the adjudication decision (Casto and White 2021, 171).

83. b Legibility deals with handwritten documents and signatures and indicates that these must be clear enough to be read. Consistent means that all documentation contains entries that are consistent and no unexplained differences of opinion in the diagnostic statements. Timely refers to the lack of a timely entry (Casto and White 2021, 193).

84. b Statements a, c, and d usually occur when a healthcare provider unknowingly or unintentionally submits an inaccurate claim for payment. Abuse generally is the result of poor medical, business, or fiscal practices (Casto and White 2021, 200).

85. c The Medicare Claims Processing Manual is one of many manuals included in the CMS Internet-Only Manuals System, which is used by the CMS program components to administer CMS programs. The CMS Program transmittals are used by CMS to communicate policies and procedures for the various payment systems' program manuals to the MACs. National coverage determinations are rules that are released by CMS that describe the circumstances under which supplies, services, or procedures are covered nationwide while local coverage determinations are used to determine coverage within the jurisdiction of a MAC rather than nationwide. The NCCI is a set of edits that was designed to promote national correct coding practices and to control improper coding that results in inappropriate payment for Part B claims (Casto and White 2021, 215).

86. d Medical conditions due to substance use, abuse, and dependence are not classified as substance-induced disorders. Assign the diagnosis code for the medical condition along with the appropriate psychoactive substance use, abuse, or dependence code. Selection of codes "in remission" requires the provider's clinical judgement. The code for MSBP is assigned to the perpetrator not the victim. The victim is assigned an appropriate code from the adult and child abuse codes (*ICD-10-CM Official Guidelines for Coding and Reporting 2022*, I.C.5.a–c).

87. d Each time a questionable service is provided, an ABN must be provided (Huey 2021, 376).

88. a An electronic health record's scheduling system often prompts the staff to do a benefits eligibility inquiry, which will identify the extent of the benefits and the amounts of copay (Handlon 2020, 246–247).

89. b Medicare beneficiaries are sent a Medicare Summary Notice which is similar to the Explanation of Benefits sent to non-Medicare Beneficiaries (Casto and White 2021, 172).

90. c The third-party payer sends an Explanation of Benefits to the patient to explain how payment on the claim was made (Casto and White 2021, 172).

91. b Each of the three RVUs is adjusted through the GPCIs to adjust for costs in different areas of the country. The national conversion factor is an across-the-board multiplier that converts the RVUs into a dollar amount. A per diem concept is not used in RBRVS. Usual and customary fees are no longer used (Casto and White 2021, 122–124).

92. d Each of the three RVUs is adjusted through the GPCIs to adjust for costs in different areas of the country. GPCIs are not relative value units (Casto and White 2021, 123).

93. b Linking informs the payer which diagnosis is associated with each procedure on the claim (Huey 2021, 376–378).

94. b When the coding professional compares the procedure description to the diagnosis description, there is a difference between the location of the foreign body; therefore, the diagnosis was not correctly linked to the procedure (Huey 2021, 376–378).

95. **b** Local Coverage Determinations provide physicians with the circumstances under which a service or procedure or supply is considered medically necessary. These apply to a MAC-wide basis rather than a nationwide basis (Casto and White 2021, 215–216).

96. **d** The denial rate is the measure that assesses the ability to comply with documentation, coding and billing requirements. The PEPPER metric is used to identify billing patterns different from the majority of other providers in the nation. The capture rate is the metric used to identify coding of secondary diagnoses. The clean claim rate assesses the ability to comply with billing edits (Casto and White 2021, 187).

97. **b** A dialysis center is considered a nonfacility in relation to the RBRVS (Casto and White 2021, 123).

CCS-P MEDICAL SCENARIOS

Exam 2 Scenario 1

DX1	S72.002D	Fracture of unspecified part of neck of left femur, subsequent encounter for closed fracture with routing healing
DX2	E11.40	Type 2 diabetes mellitus with diabetic neuropathy, unspecified
DX3	E66.9	Obesity, unspecified
DX4	L98.8	Other specified disorders of the skin and subcutaneous tissue
PR1	97162	Physical therapy evaluation; moderate complexity, require these components: a history of present problem with 1-2 personal factors and/or comorbidities that impact the plan of care; an examination of body systems using standardized tests and measures in addressing a total of 3 or more elements from any of the following: body structures and functions, activity limitations, and/or participation restrictions; an evolving clinical presentation with changing characteristics; and clinical decision making of moderate complexity using standardized patient assessment instrument and/or measurable assessment of functional outcome

Exam 2 Scenario 2

DX1	R19.7	Diarrhea, unspecified
DX2	R11.0	Nausea
DX3	S40.811A	Abrasion of right upper arm, initial encounter
DX4	S40.812A	Abrasion of left upper arm, initial encounter
PR1	99214	Office or other outpatient visit for the evaluation and management of an established patient, which requires a medically appropriate history and/or examination and moderate level of decision making
PR2	90471	Immunization administration (includes percutaneous, intradermal, subcutaneous, or intramuscular injections); 1 vaccine (single or combination vaccine/toxoid)
PR3	90714	Tetanus and diphtheria toxoid adsorbed (Td), preservative free, when administered to individuals 7 years or older, for intramuscular use

Exam 2 Scenario 3

DX1	E10.10	Type 1 diabetes mellitus with ketoacidosis, without coma
DX2	K59.00	Constipation, unspecified
PR1	99255	Inpatient consultation for a new or established patient, which requires these 3 key components: a comprehensive history, a comprehensive examination; and medical decision making of high complexity

Exam 2 Scenario 4

DX1	S76.112A	Strain of left quadriceps muscle, fascia, and tendon, initial encounter
PR1	27664	Repair, extensor tendon, leg; primary, without graft, each tendon

Exam 2 Scenario 5

DX1	C90.00	Multiple myeloma not having achieved remission
PR1	36558	Insertion of tunneled centrally inserted central venous catheter, without subcutaneous port or pump; age 5 years or older

Exam 2 Scenario 6

DX1	N18.6	End-stage renal disease
PR1	90935	Hemodialysis procedure with single evaluation by a physician or other qualified health care professional

Exam 2 Scenario 7

DX1	Q12.0	Congenital cataract
PR1	66982	Extracapsular cataract removal with insertion of intraocular lens prosthesis (1-stage procedure), manual or mechanical technique (eg, irrigation and aspiration or phacoemulsification), complex, requiring devices or techniques not generally used in routine cataract surgery (eg, iris expansion device, suture support for intraocular lens, or primary posterior capsulorrhexis) or performed on patients in the amblyogenic developmental stage; without endoscopic cyclophotocoagulation

Exam 2 Scenario 8

DX1	E10.9	Type 1 diabetes mellitus without complications
DX2	K30	Functional dyspepsia
DX3	K21.9	Gastro-esophageal reflux disease without esophagitis
PR1	91034	Esophagus, gastroesophageal reflux test; with nasal catheter pH electrode(s) placement, recording, analysis and interpretation

Exam 3

1. **d** In ICD-10-CM, mechanical complications include the mechanical breakdown/displacement, leakage, mechanical obstruction, perforation, or protrusion of the device, implant, or graft (Leon-Chisen 2022, 550–551).

2. **d** Because the patient was postoperative, the postoperative infection code (T81.40XA) should be coded, as well as a code for the cellulitis of the leg (L03.115), which identifies the specific type of postoperative infection present. Under code category T81.4-, there is a note to the coding professional to identify the infection (Optum360 2022, *ICD-10-CM Expert for Hospitals*, 1152).

3. **b** The ICD-10-CM code book defines a young primigravida as a female younger than 16 years old at time of her first delivery (Optum360 2022, *ICD-10-CM Expert for Hospitals*, Tabular List, subcategory O09.6; 875).

4. **a** A Z code would not be used because there is a specific code that more adequately describes the scenario listed (*ICD-10-CM Official Guidelines for Coding and Reporting 2022*, I.B.4).

5. **a** ICD-10-CM classifies both pathological and traumatic fractures. When coding pathological or spontaneous fractures, the fifth character identifies the specific site, and the sixth character demonstrates laterality. These fracture codes require a seventh character to identify the episode of care (Schraffenberger and Palkie 2022, 449–450).

6. **c** E10.10, E10.65, K04.7, E86.0—A diagnosis of "diabetic" ketoacidosis is coded to E10.10, Type 1 diabetes mellitus with ketoacidosis without coma. Ketoacidosis is a complication of type 1 diabetes; type 2 diabetics seldom develop ketoacidosis. A diagnosis of DKA should be classified as type 1 diabetes. The poorly controlled diabetes, abscessed tooth, and dehydration should also be coded (Leon-Chisen 2022, 165–166).

7. **b** Code assignment for HIV depends on whether the patient is symptomatic or asymptomatic. Code B20 is used for HIV that is symptomatic (Leon-Chisen 2022, 153).

8. **c** Category T31 is based on the classic "rule of nines" in estimating body surface involved: head and neck—9%; each arm—9%; each leg—18%; anterior trunk—18%; posterior trunk—18%, and genitalia—1% (Leon-Chisen 2022, 526–527).

9. **a** There are two sites to be coded—abdomen and right forearm—both second-degree burns since this was the highest level of burn for each site (*ICD-10-CM Official Guidelines for Coding and Reporting 2022*, I.C.19.d.5; Hazelwood and Venable 2014, 190).

10. **a** L89.621, L89.612—Codes from category L89, Pressure ulcer, are combination codes that identify the site of the pressure ulcer as well as the stage of the ulcer. The ICD-10-CM classifies pressure ulcer stages based on severity, which is designated by stages 1–4, unspecified stage and unstageable. Assign as many codes from category L89 as needed to identify all the pressure ulcers the patient has, if applicable (*ICD-10-CM Official Guidelines for Coding and Reporting 2022*, I.C.12.a.).

11. **d** A41.9, R65.21, J96.00—Even though the blood cultures were negative, the septicemia can be coded based on the physician's clinical findings. The signs and symptoms are not coded, only the confirmed diagnoses (*ICD-10-CM Official Guidelines for Coding and Reporting 2022*, I.C.1.d.1.a.i; *ICD-10-CM Official Guidelines for Coding and Reporting 2022*, I.C.1.d.1.b).

12. d When coding sequela, the residual condition or nature of the sequela is sequenced first, followed by the cause of the sequela (*ICD-10-CM Official Guidelines for Coding and Reporting* 2022, I.B.10).

13. c The severity of a decubitus ulcer is identified by stages I–IV. It is important to remember the definition of each of the stages so that an accurate code can be assigned (Leon-Chisen 2022, 296–297).

14. a The only reason for the admission was for the administration of radiotherapy therefore code Z51.0 is listed as the principal diagnosis with a secondary code also being listed for the pancreatic adenocarcinoma (*ICD-10-CM Official Guidelines for Coding and Reporting 2022*, 2.e.2).

15. a If the patient has a documented history of HIV and is on medication, the code for HIV (B20) is assigned. A code for the long-term use of the antiretroviral medication is also used (*ICD-10-CM Official Guidelines for Coding and Reporting 2022*, I.C.1.a.i).

16. d Confirmation of COVID-19 can be made by a positive test or by clinical documentation from a provider. If the reason for an encounter is a manifestation of COVID-19, the principal diagnosis should be COVID-19 and not the manifestation (*ICD-10-CM Official Guidelines for Coding and Reporting 2022*, I.C.1.g.1).

17. b A joint aspiration is an arthrocentesis (Huey 2021, 97–98).

18. b A removal of a portion of the patient's kidney is a partial nephrectomy (*CPT Assistant*, January 2003, 01(13): 9–21).

19. c This is an unstable finger fracture that requires manipulation but not percutaneous pinning (normally a day surgery procedure), or code 26725. In addition, the x-ray is of the fingers, not the hand, or code 73140 (*CPT Professional Edition 2022*, 187–188, 533).

20. d Tympanoplasty with mastoidectomy is coded with one code, 69641 (*CPT Assistant*, August 2008, 18(8): 4).

21. b A central venous catheter tunneled through the subclavian vein and terminated in the superior vena cava is coded as a tunneled centrally inserted central venous catheter, 36558 (*CPT Assistant*, December 2004, 12(14): 6–13).

22. d The femoral-femoral bypass is performed with material other than a vein (prosthetic graft); therefore, the correct code is 35661. Venous options are not appropriate. The thromboendarterectomy is performed on the common femoral artery. This is the illustration found at code 35371 in the (*CPT Professional Edition 2022*, 294–298).

23. a Code 62369 describes all of the work involved by the pump technician. Physician skill was not required and reprogramming was performed. Based on the coding notes found at 95991, code 62369 is the correct code (*CPT Professional Edition 2022*, 475, 812).

24. c The medial and posterior malleoli fractures are considered one type of the bimalleolar fracture of the ankle. Code 27814 describes open treatment of any of these types of fractures. The syndesmosis disruption is damaged to the joint between the tibia and fibula that often occurs with a bimalleolar or trimalleolar fracture. Code 27829 is assigned for open treatment of this disruption (Huey 2021, 98–99; *CPT Professional Edition 2022*, 202).

25. a   There are no CPT Category I codes that describe percutaneous implantation/insertion of a mitral valve. Repair of a valve is different than total replacement of a diseased/damaged valve. Category III codes were developed to describe the two approaches for this procedure. 0483T describes the percutaneous approach using a transseptal puncture (*CPT Professional Edition 2022*, 892).

26. c   The requirements for a consultation on a patient not covered by Medicare are met (Huey 2021, 330–331).

27. d   99203, 94640, 94664, J7620—This is a new patient. Since time is not documented, use the level of medical decision-making (low level) to select the code from the 99202–99205 code range. The nebulizer is 94640. The MDI teaching is 94664, and the combination of Albuterol and Atrovent is J7620, which is not coded as two individual codes (Huey 2021, 279–280, 338–341).

28. a   Code 92928 includes coronary angioplasty when performed (*CPT Professional Edition 2022*, 749–752).

29. c   The patient would be considered an established patient of the urologist, as he had received face-to-face professional services from that provider within the past three years. The physician documented the time spent with the patient, which would be used to select the appropriate code from the established patient code range (99211–99215) (Huey 2021, 338–341).

30. c   The documentation supports the detailed level of history. There is a chief complaint (cold), an extended HPI (four elements: quality, location, associated signs and symptoms, and duration), an extended review of systems (two elements: respiratory and constitutional), and a pertinent past, family, and social history (no chronic conditions) (Huey 2021, 314–316).

31. c   Modifiers LT and RT are used to describe that x-rays are performed on each side (Huey 2021, 233).

32. c   According to the Coding Guidelines, modifier 26 is required because the pathologist is not employed by the facility and is billing separately. Each specimen must be reported separately (*CPT Professional Edition 2022*, 688–690; Huey 2021, 251–252).

33. d   Code 31646 specifically describes a subsequent bronchoscopy with therapeutic aspiration during the same hospital stay. Coding a different bronchoscopy code with modifier 76 is inappropriate (*CPT Professional Edition 2022*, 229).

34. b   The coding notes prior to code 99495 identify that the patient must have an interactive contact within 2 business days of the hospital discharge. TCM series cannot be billed following discharge from a skilled nursing facility or when the patient is discharged to a skilled nursing facility and the face-to-face visit is required within 7 to 14 days, based on the type of decision-making required (*CPT Professional Edition 2022*, 71–72).

35. d   Codes from the wound debridement subsection are reported by the deepest level of tissue removed. Wounds debrided at the same depth should be added together (*CPT Professional Edition 2022*, 95–97).

36. d   A surgical sinus endoscopy always includes both a diagnostic sinus endoscopy and a sinusotomy (Huey 2021, 112).

37. d When reporting multiple infusions, only one "initial" service should be reported. For physician reporting, the "initial" service is the "key or primary reason for the encounter." In this case, the patient came into the physician's office for chemotherapy. Code 96361 should be used to report the hydration, indicating that it is secondary or subsequent service (*CPT Professional Edition 2022*, 822–828).

38. a Lacerations of the same site grouping and same complexity are added together for coding with the most complex repair listed first (*CPT Professional Edition 2022*, 106–109).

39. c Codes for excision of lesions include simple closure, so it would not be coded separately. Each lesion excised must be reported separately (*CPT Professional Edition 2022*, 101–105).

40. a The CPT code book defines a consultation as a type of service provided by a physician at the request of another physician or appropriate source to either recommend care for a specific condition or problem or to determine whether to accept responsibility for ongoing management of the patient's care. Modifier 57 is to be used when an E/M service was the result of an initial decision to perform surgery on a patient (Huey 2021, 57).

41. b According to the National Correct Coding Initiative (NCCI), since the entire lobe was removed during the same operative episode, the biopsy is not separately reportable (CMS 2021b).

42. a According to the National Correct Coding Initiative (NCCI), bilateral codes may not be unbundled into two unilateral codes, nor may they be reported with two units of service (CMS 2021b).

43. c The patient would be considered an established patient since she regularly sees this physician. Medical decision-making is at a low level, based on the number and complexity of problems addressed and risk of complications and morbidity (*CPT Professional Edition 2022*, 16–18).

44. d Because the lesion extends into the soft tissue of the back, it must be coded from the musculoskeletal system subsection, not integumentary (Smith 2021, 79).

45. d If only a portion of the lesion is removed, the breast biopsy is considered incisional. When the entire lesion is removed, the procedure is classified as an excision of a breast lesion (Huey 2021, 88–89).

46. b Vancomycin is an antibiotic, so the infusion would be coded from the section on therapeutic, prophylactic, and diagnostic injections and infusions (*CPT Professional Edition 2022*, 822–826).

47. c Because the biopsies are performed during colonoscopy, the combination code for colonoscopy with biopsy must be used. There was no mention of hot biopsy forceps (*CPT Professional Edition 2022*, 380–381)

48. d THD involves the use of a special model of anoscope combined with Doppler radar to perform the procedure described. Code 46948 was added in 2020 to report this technique (Smith 2021, 149).

49. a According to the Surgery Guidelines, the consultation to determine the need for the procedure is always excluded from the surgical global (*CPT Professional Edition 2022*, 88).

50. d   Assign a code from category I16, Hypertensive crisis, for documented hypertensive urgency, hypertensive emergency, or unspecified hypertensive crisis. Code also any identified hypertensive disease (I10–I15). The sequencing is based on the reason for the encounter (*ICD-10-CM Official Guidelines for Coding and Reporting 2022*, 1.C.9.a.10).

51. b   Patient may have several chronic conditions that coexist at the time of hospital admission and qualify as additional diagnoses. If there is documentation in the health record to indicate the patient has a chronic condition, it should be coded. Chronic diseases treated on an ongoing basis may be coded and reported as many times as the patient receives treatment and care for the condition(s) (*ICD-10-CM Official Guidelines for Coding and Reporting 2022*, Section IV: Diagnostic Coding and Reporting Guidelines for Outpatient Services).

52. b   Linking informs the payer which diagnosis is associated with each procedure on the claim (Huey 2021, 376–378).

53. d   The Official Documentation Guidelines clarify the assignment of E/M codes by describing the necessary elements in great detail. Standardized definitions are set for different levels of history, examination, and medical decision-making (Huey 2021, 310–311).

54. d   If the drug is provided by the provider, the coding professional should consult the list of HCPCS Level II National Codes to locate the code (J code) for the specific drug administered at the appropriate dose (Huey 2021, 283–286).

55. d   Dr. Smith would charge for all of the antenatal services. Dr. Jones would assign code 59410 to report delivery of the baby, expressing the placenta, and providing all the postpartum care. This is all covered by code 59410. It is not correct to use two codes for the delivery only and the postpartum care only (59409 and 59430). It is also incorrect to code the delivery of the placenta if it is part of the delivery. Modifier 52 added to the total delivery code is not appropriate to use (*CPT Professional Edition 2022*, 450–453).

56. c   This query is leading the physician to aspiration pneumonia as a diagnosis (Handlon 2020, 289–290).

57. b   This is the only statement that is not true about the query. This query is nonleading and multiple choice is an appropriate format (Handlon 2020, 289–290).

58. b   The query gives the clinical indicators and asks the physician to specify the type of chronic heart failure. Choices a and c are leading queries (Handlon 2020, 289–290).

59. a   The histology of a neoplasm identifies the structure of the cells and the tissue that comprises the tumor new growth. The histology of tissue is determined by a pathologist and documented in the pathology report (Reynolds and Morey 2020, 115).

60. c   Progress notes are chronological statements about the patient's response to treatment during his or her stay at the facility (Reynolds and Morey 2020, 113).

61. a   The pneumonia and earlier bunionectomy have no bearing on the current admission (Leon-Chisen 2022, 28–31).

62. d   Abnormal findings from laboratory results are not coded and reported unless the physician indicates their clinical significance. If the findings are outside the normal range and the physician has ordered other tests to evaluate the condition or has prescribed treatment, it is appropriate to ask the physician whether the diagnosis code(s) for the abnormal findings should be added (*ICD-10-CM Official Guidelines for Coding and Reporting 2022* III.B).

63. d   The OIG sets forth an annual work plan (Bowman 2017, 459).

64. a   Providers who voluntarily report fraudulent conduct need to use the Provider Self-Disclosure Protocol form (Bowman 2017, 461).

65. c   The record would be considered incomplete if all progress notes were not signed at discharge. If the progress notes in the incomplete record are not signed within the specified time frame specified in the medical staff bylaws, the record is considered delinquent (Reynolds and Morey 2020, 128).

66. a   In ICD-10-CM, hypersensitivities or allergic reactions that occur as qualitatively different responses to a drug, which are acquired only after re-exposure to the drug is the definition of an adverse effect (Leon-Chisen 2022, 532–534).

67. b   If a patient admitted with glaucoma and the stage progresses during the admission, assign the code for the highest stage documented (*ICD-10-CM Official Guidelines for Coding and Reporting 2022*, I.C.7.a.4).

68. c   Patients who have undergone kidney transplant may still have some form of chronic kidney disease because the kidney transplant may not fully restore kidney function. Code T86.10 should be assigned for documented complications of a kidney transplant, such as failure or rejection. It should not be assigned for post kidney transplant patients who have CKD unless a transplant complication such as transplant failure or rejection is documented (*ICD-10-CM Official Guidelines for Coding and Reporting 2022*, I.C.14.a.2).

69. b   HCCs are only valid for one year as documenting these on at least a yearly basis encourages traditional managed care concepts (Watson 2018, 50).

70. d   ICD-10-PCS procedure codes are not used to determine a patient's RAF. Patient's age and gender are considered demographic characteristics and are used to determine the RAF as are ICD-10-CM diagnosis codes (Watson 2018, 46).

71. c   The HIPAA Privacy Rule recognizes and incorporates the principle of "minimum necessary." Generally, only the minimum necessary amount of information necessary to fulfill the purpose of the request should be shared with internal users and external requestors (Brinda and Watters 2020, 318).

72. d   The HIPAA Privacy Rule does not provide access to the patient for the following: oral information, psychotherapy notes, and information compiled in anticipation of, or for use in, a civil, criminal, or administrative action or proceeding (Brinda and Watters 2020, 323).

73. b   While the Privacy Rule applies to all PHI, the Security Rule applies only to PHI transmitted or maintained in electronic form (Reynolds and Brodnik 2017, 265).

74. a   Security awareness training is required by the Security Rule as an administrative safeguard (Reynolds and Brodnik 2017, 273).

75. b   Per *Coding Clinic* advice, the code for the pulmonary embolism is coded as principal diagnosis with an additional code for the fact that it is a sequela of the previous COVID infection. Because the patient no longer has COVID, the code U09.9 is appropriate to use (*AHA Coding Clinic* Fourth Quarter 2021, 101–110).

76. d   The patient does not currently have COVID-19 but the history of infectious disease demonstrates that she did have it in the past. The main reason for the encounter was a follow-up to her previous condition. Her diabetes mellitus is also coded as it is evaluated and is a chronic condition (*ICD-10-CM Official Guidelines for Coding and Reporting 2022,* 1.C.1.g).

77. a   When the physician performs a service in an ambulatory surgical center, it should be billed as "facility" place of service (Casto and White 2021, 123).

78. d   The final decision in selecting the setting is a blend of the above factors (Casto and White 2021, 123).

79. c   Because the physician is out of town, this would not be considered as "incident to." Therefore, the claim is submitted under the APRN's NPI (Casto and White 2021, 125–126).

80. a   The third visit can be billed "incident to" (under the physician's provider number) because the "incident to" criteria was met: The service was provided in the physician's office—The physician was on premises (direct supervision)—An employee of the physician provided the service—The service was part of the treatment plan initiated by the physician (Casto and White 2021, 125–126).

81. c   The CERT program measures improper payments in various healthcare settings for Medicare. The purpose of CERT is to measure improper payments, not to measure fraud (Casto and White 2021, 203).

82. b   Upcoding is the fraudulent process of submitting codes for reimbursement that indicate more complex or higher-paying services than the patient actually received. Unbundling and exploding deals with the process in which individual component codes are submitted for reimbursement rather than a single comprehensive code. Optimizing generally refers to getting the appropriate reimbursement based on documentation (Casto and White 2021, 202).

83. b   The Medicare Claims Processing Manual is one of many manuals included in the CMS Internet-Only Manuals System, which is used by the CMS program components to administer CMS programs. The CMS Program transmittals are used by CMS to communicate policies and procedures for the various payment systems' program manuals to the MACs. National coverage determinations are rules that are released by CMS that describe the circumstances under which supplies, services, or procedures are covered nationwide while local coverage determinations are used to determine coverage within the jurisdiction of a MAC rather than nationwide. The NCCI is a set of edits that was designed to promote national correct coding practices and to control improper coding that results in inappropriate payment for Part B claims (Casto and White 2021, 215).

84. d   In the systematic random sampling technique, the medical records used for the audit are identified by selecting every nth unit on the list. An example is taking a list of medical records for the month of January and selecting the first record and then every sixth record thereafter (Casto and White 2021, 211).

85. b   In the weighted code over code methodology, select categories of codes, such as the first-listed or principal diagnosis codes are given a greater weight than other codes. The greater the assigned weight, the greater emphasis the facility places on the correct assignment of the code. In the code over code, all codes are assigned an equal weight. Emphasis is placed on the correct assignment of each code (Casto and White 2021, 210).

86. c   A clinical validation denial indicates that there is insufficient clinical indicators or discussion points within the medical record documentation to support the diagnosis assigned to the patient. External auditors examine the medical record documentation to assess if a patient's disease or condition is appropriately supported by clinical evaluation, treatment, diagnostic procedures, increased nursing care, or extended length of stay (Casto and White 2021, 219).

87. c   Disclosure for HIPAA requirements is not listed as a main purpose of clinical documentation (Hunt and Kirk 2020, 266–267).

88. b   The goal in claims submittal is to submit each claim as a clean claim, which means it contains all of the required and accurate information. A clean claim is essential in order to receive timely and accurate reimbursement (Huey 2021, 382–383).

89. a   Electronic funds transfer or EFT indicates that reimbursement payments are sent electronically to providers' banks (Casto and White 2021, 173–174).

90. d   The EOB, RA, and MSN can all be used in the reconciliation process. The Outpatient Code Editor is used to scrub claims for errors (Casto and White 2021, 217–218).

91. c   For Medicare, a nonparticipating physician who does not accept assignment may not bill the patient more than the Medicare limiting charge, which is 115 percent of the Medicare approved amount (Huey 2021, 371).

92. d   CMS will reimburse the physician for 80 percent of the Medicare Fee Schedule Amount, which is $200.00. $200.00 × .80 = $160.00. The Medicare beneficiary is responsible for the remaining 20 percent (Casto and White 2021, 125–126).

93. c   The patient has a recurrent inguinal hernia and this is captured in the diagnosis code (Schraffenberger and Palkie 2022, 385–386; *CPT Assistant* Nov. 1999, 24; March 2000, 9).

94. d   When the coding professional compares the procedure description to the diagnosis description, there is a difference between the type of immunization being coded and the shoulder pain is linked to the cholesterol. Therefore, the diagnosis was not correctly linked to the procedure (Huey 2021, 376–378).

95. b   The diagnosis code does not prove medical necessity for placement of a pacemaker. No additional CPT codes are needed as the insertion of the electrode is included in 33206 (Handlon 2020, 247).

96. a The denial rate is the measure that assesses the ability to comply with documentation, coding, and billing requirements. The PEPPER metric is used to identify billing patterns different from the majority of other providers in the nation. The capture rate is the metric used to identify coding of secondary diagnoses. The clean claim rate assesses the ability to comply with billing edits (Casto and White 2021, 187).

97. c Under RBRVS, anesthesia services have a separate payment method based on base units and time units. There is also a separate conversion factor adjusted for locality (Casto and White 2021, 125).

CCS-P MEDICAL SCENARIOS

Exam 3 Scenario 1

DX1	A41.59	Other Gram-negative sepsis
DX2	N39.0	Urinary tract infection site not specified
DX3	B96.89	Other specified bacterial agents as the cause of diseases classified elsewhere
PR1	99253	Inpatient consultation for a new or established patient, which requires these 3 key components: a detailed history; a detailed examination; and medical decision making of low complexity

Exam 3 Scenario 2

DX1	S22.42XA	Multiple fractures of ribs, left side, initial encounter for closed fracture
DX2	S27.321A	Contusion of lung, unilateral, initial encounter
DX3	S27.2XXA	Traumatic hemopneumothorax, initial encounter
DX4	S32.502A	Unspecified fracture of left pubis, initial encounter for closed fracture
PR1	99223	Initial hospital care, per day, for the evaluation and management of a patient, which requires these 3 key components: a comprehensive history; a comprehensive examination; and medical decision making of high complexity

Exam 3 Scenario 3

DX1	E26.01	Conn's syndrome
DX2	D35.02	Benign neoplasm of left adrenal gland
DX3	I10	Essential (primary) hypertension
DX4	E87.6	Hypokalemia
PR1	60650	Laparoscopy, surgical, with adrenalectomy, partial or complete, or exploration of adrenal gland with or without biopsy, transabdominal, lumbar or dorsal

Exam 3 Scenario 4

DX1	D05.11	Intraductal carcinoma in situ of right breast
PR1	19302	Mastectomy, partial (eg, lumpectomy, tylectomy, quadrantectomy, segmentectomy); with axillary lymphadenectomy

Exam 3 Scenario 5

DX1	J30.81	Allergic rhinitis due to animal (cat) (dog) hair and dander
DX2	J30.1	Allergic rhinitis due to pollen
PR1	95125	Professional services for allergen immunotherapy in the office or institution of the prescribing physician or other qualified health care professional, including provision of allergenic extract: 2 or more injections

Exam 3 Scenario 6

DX1	I25.10	Atherosclerotic heart disease of native coronary artery without angina pectoris
PR1	93453	Combined right and left heart catheterization including intraprocedural injection(s) for left ventriculography, imaging supervision and interpretation, when performed

Exam 3 Scenario 7

DX1	Q40.0	Congenital hypertrophic pyloric stenosis
DX2	Q89.09	Congenital malformations of spleen
PR1	38120	Laparoscopy, surgical, splenectomy
PR2	43659	Unlisted laparoscopic procedure, stomach

Exam 3 Scenario 8

DX1	L03.116	Cellulitis, of left lower limb
DX2	E11.51	Type 2 diabetes mellitus with diabetic peripheral angiopathy without gangrene
PR1	99214	Office or other outpatient visit for the evaluation and management of an established patient, which requires a medically appropriate history and/or examination and moderate level of medical decision making
PR2	96374	Therapeutic, prophylactic, or diagnostic injection (specify substance or drug); intravenous push, single or initial substance/drug
PR3	J0696	Injection, ceftriaxone sodium, per 250 mg
PR4	J0696	Injection, ceftriaxone sodium, per 250 mg
PR5	J0696	Injection, ceftriaxone sodium, per 250 mg
PR6	J0696	Injection, ceftriaxone sodium, per 250 mg

Exam 4

1. a   This occasion of service was only for the radiation therapy; therefore, it is sequenced before the code for the neoplasm (*ICD-10-CM Official Guidelines for Coding and Reporting 2022*, I.C.2.e.2).

2. b   In ICD-10-CM, alcohol dependence is classified to subcategory F10.2 with the fifth character of this subcategory specifying the presence of intoxication, intoxication delirium, alcohol-induced mood disorder, psychotic disorder, and other alcohol-induced disorders (Leon-Chisen 2022, 184–185).

3. b   The primary diagnosis is the pernicious anemia with the agammaglobulinemia, and gastritis being associated with the anemia and therefore placed after the anemia code (Schraffenberger and Palkie 2022, 174).

4. b   Cellulitis is not a sequela of an injury (Schraffenberger and Palkie 2022, 400–401).

5. a   B26.9—The signs and symptoms are not coded. Infectious parotitis is classified as mumps (Schraffenberger and Palkie 2022, 554–556).

6. c   T45.511A, T39.011A, R31.9—Coumadin with an over-the-counter drug not prescribed by the physician is considered a poisoning. The hematuria is also coded (Leon-Chisen 2022, 532–534).

7. d   The *Official Guidelines* state that the code for the underlying cause (infection or trauma) must be sequenced first (*ICD-10-CM Official Guidelines for Coding and Reporting 2022*, I.C.1.d.1.a; I.C.1.d.1.b).

8. b   This code is used because there was no mention of hemorrhage or perforation and was also without obstruction (Schraffenberger and Palkie 2022, 382–383).

9. c   When a patient has bilateral glaucoma and each eye is documented as having a different type or stage, and the classification distinguishes laterality, assign the appropriate code for each eye rather than the code for bilateral glaucoma (*ICD-10-CM Official Guidelines for Coding and Reporting 2022*, 1.C.7.a.3).

10. c   The pain associated with the migraine would not be coded and there is a symptom code for the abdominal pain and the chest pain. Category G89 can be used to code neoplasm related pain (Schraffenberger and Palkie 2022, 245–247).

11. a   When two or more sites are described as "metastatic" in the physician's documentation, each of the sites would be coded as secondary or metastatic. A code would also be assigned to the primary site, if known, or coded to C80.1 when it is not known (Leon-Chisen 2022, 469–470).

12. a   When the treatment is directed toward the secondary site only, the secondary neoplasm is listed as the principal or principal diagnosis even if the primary malignancy is still present (*ICD-10-CM Official Guidelines for Coding and Reporting 2022*, I.C.2.b).

13. c   The physician has not documented this as complication of the surgery and the weakness and low blood pressure are symptoms (Schraffenberger and Palkie 2022, 98).

14. a   The ICD-10-CM coding guideline for hypertensive heart and chronic kidney disease states "Assign codes from combination category I13, Hypertensive heart and chronic kidney disease, when both hypertensive kidney disease and hypertensive heart disease are stated in the diagnosis. Assume a relationship between the hypertension and the chronic kidney disease whether or not the condition is designated. If heart failure is present, assign an additional code from category I50 to identify the type of heart failure. The appropriate code from category N18, Chronic kidney disease, should be used as a secondary code with a code from category I13 to identify the stage of chronic kidney disease." Additionally, a code should also be assigned for the diabetic polyneuropathy (*ICD-10-CM Official Guidelines for Coding and Reporting 2022*, I.C.9.a.3).

15. a   The diagnosis states that it was an accidental poisoning therefore the correct ICD-10-CM code is T40.2X1A (Schraffenberger and Palkie 2022, 615–617).

16. b   Pre-existing hypertension is always considered to be a complicating factor in pregnancy, childbirth, or the puerperium and is classified in category O10, Pre-existing hypertension complicating pregnancy, childbirth, and the puerperium. Code O10.013 is assigned to report pre-existing benign essential hypertension when the patient is in the third trimester. A note in the Tabular at the beginning of Chapter 15 defines the third trimester as 28 weeks, 0 days until delivery. An additional code to identify the weeks of gestation is also assigned. An additional note at the beginning of Chapter 15 states to use an additional code from category Z3A, Weeks of gestation, to identify the specific week of the pregnancy (Schraffenberger and Palkie 2022, 494, 506–507).

17. c   The excised diameter calculation is displayed on page 101 of the *CPT Professional Edition* (*CPT Professional Edition 2022*, 101–102; Huey 2021, 80–81).

18. c   One combination code is required to describe the angiography along with the left heart catheterization (Huey 2021, 272–273; *CPT Professional Edition 2022*, 764–773).

19. a   All of the work described is included in code 29881 (Huey 2021, 105–106).

20. c   Removal of the leads is coded separately from the insertion of the new leads (*CPT Assistant*, Summer 1994, 02(4): 10–26).

21. b   The abscess is aspirated through a burr hole, described by CPT code 61150. The stereotactic guidance is coded as 61781 because the abscess is of the brain, or intradural, meaning inside the dura layer (in the brain), indexed under Drainage, abscess, brain (*CPT Assistant*, July 2011, 21(7): 12; *CPT Professional Edition 2022*, 460, 467).

22. c   Code 33274 includes device evaluation (*CPT Professional Edition 2022*, 248–255).

23. d   This procedure is performed using a laparoscopic approach, therefore either 58545 or 58546 could be the correct answer. However, only 58546 describes the removal of seven intramural myomas, even if the total weight is not over 250 g (*CPT Assistant*, January 2004, 01(14): 26).

24. b   The repair of the ruptured spleen is coded as 38115 because the code description states "with or without partial splenectomy" (*CPT Assistant*, Summer 1993, 02(3): 5–12).

25. a   50365, 49422—Code 50365 includes the recipient nephrectomy and all the anastomoses required to transplant the kidney. The peritoneal dialysis catheter is a tunneled catheter and its removal is coded with 49422 (*CPT Assistant*, April 2005, 15(4): 10–12).

26. c   New patient and established patient definitions do not apply to emergency department evaluation and management codes. It is necessary that the three key components are described. Time is not an issue in emergency department coding, and any physician can use these codes (Huey 2021, 332).

27. c   The documentation states that the laceration was closed with one simple stitch. This does not support the assignment of the code for a complex repair that was listed on the encounter summary (*CPT Professional Edition 2022*, 106–109).

28. c   Refer to the chart in CPT to see that 115 minutes of critical care is coded using three codes (*CPT Professional Edition 2022*, 32–33).

29. b   Modifier 25 should be assigned to the E/M code if a significant, separately identifiable E/M service is performed by the same physician on the same day as a procedure (Huey 2021, 55).

30. b   Since the physician documented 45 minutes with the patient, time can be used to select a code from the established patient code range (99211–99215) (Huey 2021, 338–341).

31. c   If a diagnostic colonoscopy is discontinued before the scope reaches the splenic flexure, it is coded as a sigmoidoscopy (*CPT Professional Edition 2022*, 381).

32. b   Modifiers would not be appended to unlisted codes because these codes describe new or unclassified procedures that have no standard description. Therefore, the description does not need to be modified (Huey 2021, 54).

33. c   Modifier 76 is used to indicate that a procedure is repeated by the same physician on the same day (Huey 2021, 59).

34. d   Modifier 79 is appended to the second procedure to indicate that an unrelated procedure by the same physician or other qualified healthcare professional was performed during the postoperative period of the open treatment of the femoral fracture (*CPT Professional Edition 2022*, 919).

35. b   The location of the donor site is not needed to code grafts as the harvesting of the graft is included in the graft code. However, if the donor site requires skin grafting or local flaps, an additional code would be reported (Huey 2021, 85).

36. d   The patient receives 600 mg of Rocephin. The HCPCS code description for J0696 is 250 mg. Therefore, 3 units of Rocephin must be reported (250 mg, 250 mg, and some of the third unit of 250 mg) (Huey 2021, 285–284).

37. d   Replacement casts are coded separately (*CPT Professional Edition 2022*, 210; Huey 2021, 104).

38. b   The procedure described is a colonoscopy with biopsy and is coded as 45380 (Huey 2021, 145–146).

39. c   Because the patient is an inpatient, a code should be selected from the Subsequent Hospital Care subsection of the E/M section (99231–99233) (*CPT Professional Edition 2022*, 24–25).

40. c   Unbundling is the practice of coding services separately that should be coded together as a package because all parts are included within one code and therefore one price. Unbundling done deliberately could be considered fraud (Huey 2021, 409).

41. c   A laparoscopic-assisted vaginal hysterectomy is referred to as a Laparoscopy, surgical, with vaginal hysterectomy in CPT. The code is determined based on whether the uterus is under or over 250 grams and where the tubes and ovaries are removed at the same session. An additional code for the salpingo-oophorectomy should not be assigned (Huey 2021, 173–174).

42. c   According to the National Correct Coding initiative (NCCI), in this situation, the anesthesia service may be reported by the second provider (CMS 2021b).

43. d   Using medical decision-making to support coding, the correct code is 99214. The number and complexity of problems to be addressed is moderate, as is the amount and or complexity of data to be reviewed and analyzed, and the risk (Huey 2021, 339–341).

44. b   The code for reporting prolonged service can be assigned if the coding professional is using time as the basis for assigning the E/M code, and the minimum time in the code description has been exceeded by 15 minutes. A helpful table on page 44 of *CPT Professional Edition* guides the coding professional in code selection (Huey 2021, 337–339; *CPT Professional Edition* 2022, 43–44).

45. c   The description of code 59812 describes surgical treatment of an incomplete abortion. The code description for 58120 clearly states that the D&C is nonobstetrical. There was no conization of the cervix, and the abortion was not induced (Huey 2021, 179).

46. b   A fine needle aspiration is performed with a fine needle, whereas a core needle biopsy is performed with a larger bore needle. There is no mention of excision of the lesion (Huey 2021, 77–78).

47. c   When a physician uses the term "myringotomy" for insertion of ventilating tubes, it is coded as tympanostomy. Notes beneath the code instruct the coding professional to use modifier 50 for bilateral procedure (Huey 2021, 200–201; *CPT Professional Edition 2022*, 517).

48. d   When a patient is admitted to the hospital on the same day as an outpatient visit, code only the admission. If a patient is admitted and discharged on the same day, a code from the "Observation or Inpatient care Services (Including Admission and Discharge Services)" must be used (Huey 2021, 328–329).

49. a   Healthcare Common Procedural Coding System (HCPCS) codes are used to code procedures that are not covered in the CPT book. These codes should be consulted to choose the correct answer (CMS 2022).

50. c   The *ICD-10-CM Official Guidelines for Coding and Reporting 2022*, Section IV, subpart H, Diagnostic Coding and Reporting Guidelines for Outpatient Services indicate that when a physician qualifies a diagnostic statement as "probable," the condition qualified with that statement should not be coded as if it existed. Rather, the condition should be coded to the highest level of certainty such as the signs and symptoms the patient exhibits. The history of cholecystectomy has no relevance to the current encounter and should not be coded per the *ICD-10-CM Official Guidelines for Coding and Reporting 2022*, Section IV: Code All Documented Conditions That Coexist, subpart J.

51. b Since the colonoscope reached the terminal ileum the procedure would be coded as a colonoscopy (not sigmoidoscopy). Because the procedure indications included a personal history of polyps and a family history of colon cancer, the procedure would be coded as a screening colonoscopy, G0105 (Smith 2021, 144).

52. b The *Official ICD-10-CM Coding Guidelines* are published annually in *Coding Clinic*, which is published by the Central Office on ICD-10-CM Coding of the American Hospital Association (*AHA Coding Clinic* Third Quarter 2021, 3–4).

53. c LCDs and NCDs are very important in establishing medical necessity. When medical necessity is in question, an ABN should be completed. Encoders and groupers do not assist in establishing medical necessity (Schraffenberger and Palkie 2022, 726–727).

54. a CMS developed a list of coding edits known as the NCCI to prevent inappropriate unbundling of related services (Huey 2021, 433).

55. a If the gastroenteritis and colitis is not specified as infective, the default code is noninfective. Although there is an Excludes 1 note that references the diarrhea code, R19.7, it is not necessary to code this as it is a symptom of colitis and thus only code K52.9 should be coded (*AHA Coding Clinic* Third Quarter 2021, 3–4).

56. c In scenario a the patient was asymptomatic and no further evaluation or treatment was carried out. In scenario b the cardiomegaly was an isolated finding, which had no implications for the patient's care. In scenario d physician documentation is adequate to diagnose sepsis (Leon-Chisen 2022, 28–31).

57. a Documentation that is consistent does not contradict itself. Documentation that is precise is clearly defined and reliable documentation is trustworthy. Complete documentation is detailed and has maximum content fully addressing all concerns in the record (Handlon 2020, 287).

58. d The goal of physician queries is to document with specificity and accuracy. Reimbursement impact should not be the goal of queries. Coding professionals are not qualified to diagnose patients or perform procedures (Handlon 2020, 287–288).

59. c The diagnosis of hypercholesterolemia is to be sequenced first, followed by the obesity (Schraffenberger and Palkie 2022, 202).

60. d Code J01.80 is the correct answer. This code is used when more than one sinus is involved (Optum360 2022, *ICD-10-CM Expert for Hospitals*, Alphabetic Index, main term Sinusitis).

61. b LEEP is a loop electrode excision procedure. If the procedure involves removal of a cone-shaped portion of the cervix (conization), it will be coded as 57461. If it involves only loop electrode biopsy of the cervix, it would be coded as 57460 (Huey 2021, 172).

62. c This is a preventive medicine visit, coded based on age. Vaccines were administered after counseling to patient of age 6, therefore, the 90460–90461 series of administration codes are used (Huey 2021, 264–266).

63. d By definition, this describes upcoding. This practice puts an organization or provider at risk of violating federal and state laws (Hunt and Kirk 2020, 296).

64. a   By definition, this describes optimization. Clinical documentation improvement and coding compliance programs support coding optimization (Hunt and Kirk 2020, 296).

65. b   In order to assign a consultation code, the documentation must include the need and request for consultation, and signed report of the consultant must be provided to the referring physician. Consulting physicians do not assume *responsibility* for the patient's care (*CPT Professional Edition 2022*, 27–28).

66. c   The immunization administration code is missing from the list of codes. Immunization administration must be coded along with the vaccine (*CPT Professional Edition 2022*, 720).

67. a   J15.212, Z22.322—When the patient has a MRSA infection and the physician documents MRSA colonization, both codes can be used (*ICD-10-CM Official Guidelines for Coding and Reporting 2022*, I.C.1.e.1.a–c).

68. c   Reliability refers to the consistency of any data set (LeBlanc 2020, 702).

69. a   Acute respiratory infection would be not included. The CMS-HCC model does not include acute illnesses and injuries that are not predictive of ongoing healthcare costs. A review of HCCs shows that metastatic cancers, lymphoma, and stroke are included (Watson 2018, 47–48.)

70. c   CMS-HCCs are used to risk adjust for the Medicare Advantage programs. The RxHCC is used for health plan prescription rates, the HHS-HCCs for the Affordable Care Act Health Plan Premiums, and the 3M-APR-DRGs are used in US News Rankings (Watson 2018, 46).

71. b   Disclosures used for treatment do not need to be disclosed (Rinehart-Thompson 2017a, 224).

72. b   A covered entity's documentation related to the Privacy and Security Rules must be retained for six years from its date of creation, or the date in which it was last in effect, whichever is later (Reynolds and Brodnik 2017, 279).

73. c   A significant threshold is considered 500 affected people. If 500 or more people are affected by the breach, the secretary of HHS is to be notified immediately (Rinehart-Thompson 2017b, 250).

74. d   A red flag is a pattern, practice, or specific activity that may indicate identity theft. Red flags should be used as triggers to identify possible identity theft (Olenik and Reynolds 2017, 291).

75. b   A cast application is included in the closed treatment of the trimalleolar ankle fracture. Correction of the diagnosis code would validate coding for the cast application. A cast application is included in the closed treatment of the trimalleolar ankle fracture (*CPT Professional Edition 2022*, 210).

76. d   The place where critical care is offered is not a factor in billing for critical care; time spent by nurses is not included in critical care time; only one physician may bill for critical care services during any one single period of time even if more than one physician is providing care to a critically ill patient. Procedures (such as CPR) that are not included in critical care services may be reported separately (CMS 2021a).

77. c   The correct formula for a "nonfacility" is $8.26 \times 1 + 4.99 \times .889 + .99 \times .707 = 13.3960$ (Casto and White 2021, 122–123).

78. a   This is considered a nonfacility so the correct formula is: $6.71 \times 1.032 + 17.48 \times 1.130 + .78 \times .607 = 27.1505 \times \$36.88 = \$1,001.31$ (Casto and White 2021, 122–123).

79. b   The NP's work is considered as "incident to" the physician's plan of care so all visits can be billed under the physician's NPI (Casto and White 2021, 125–126).

80. b   This is an example of "incident to" billing and will be billed under the surgeon's NPI (Casto and White 2021, 125–126).

81. b   The Medicare Claims Processing Manual is one of many manuals included in the CMS Internet-Only Manuals System, which is used by the CMS program components to administer CMS programs. The CMS Program transmittals are used by CMS to communicate policies and procedures for the various payment systems' program manuals to the MACs. National coverage determinations are rules that are released by CMS that describe the circumstances under which supplies, services, or procedures are covered nationwide while local coverage determinations are used to determine coverage within the jurisdiction of a MAC rather than nationwide. The NCCI is a set of edits that was designed to promote national correct coding practices and to control improper coding that results in inappropriate payment for Part B claims (Casto and White 2021, 215).

82. d   Answer choices a, b, and c are all types of claim denials. There is no ancillary service denial (Casto and White 2021, 219).

83. a   In 1991, the OIG released seven elements that the office believed should serve as the foundation of an effective corporate compliance plan. The OIG is a division of the Department of Health and Human Services that investigates issues of noncompliance in the Medicare and Medicaid programs, such as fraud and abuse (Casto and White 2021, 200).

84. d   Laterality may be based on medical record documentation from other clinicians if the patient's provider does not document it. If the laterality is not stated, assign the code for the unspecified side. If there is a code for "bilateral," two codes are not needed to code right and left sides (*ICD-10-CM Official Guidelines for Coding and Reporting 2022*, I.B.13).

85. c   Alcohol-related disorders must be documented by the patient's provider but the other conditions may be documented by other clinicians involved in the care of the patient (*ICD-10-CM Official Guidelines for Coding and Reporting 2022*, I.B).

86. a   Code Z20.822 is used for patients with both actual and suspected exposure to COVID-19 so b is incorrect. For an asymptomatic who tests positive for COVID-19, they are assigned code U07.1. For patients with a history of COVID-19, they are assigned code Z86.16, Personal history of COVID-19 (*ICD-10-CM Official Guidelines for Coding and Reporting 2022*, I.C.1.g).

87. c   The charge summary is sometimes called the office service report and contains a summary of all billing data entered for the practice on one day (Huey 2021, 398–401).

88. c   Medicare typically doesn't cover preventive medicine, but a new benefit was provided in The Medicare Prescription Drug, Improvement, and Modernization Act of 2003 that provides one preventive physical examination, or the "Welcome to Medicare Physical," for new Medicare Part B enrollees within the first 12 months of entitlement (Huey 2021, 346).

89. b The front-end processes cause the largest percent of denials with eligibility and registration being the most significant reasons (Handlon 2020, 264).

90. a LCDs are used to determine coverage on a MAC-wide basis while NCDs are used to determine coverage on a nationwide basis. Medicare Claims Processing Manuals describe administrative functions such as operating instructions, policies and procedures on statutes, regulations, and guidelines. Program transmittals are used by CMS to communicate policies and procedures on various prospective payment systems (Casto and White 2021, 215).

91. d A non-PAR who accepts assignment is given a 5 percent reduction from what a PAR would receive. Therefore, the physician would receive (from the CMS and the patient) $190.00. The CMS portion is 80 percent of that amount or $152.00 (Casto and White 2021, 125–126).

92. c Anesthesiologists have a separate payment system that uses base units and time units to determine payment. There is also a unique conversion factor for anesthesiologists (Casto and White 2021, 125–126).

93. d All of the above are considered as common forms of fraud and abuse except for failing to have a compliance officer in the facility (Casto and White 2021, 200).

94. a During the pre-registration process, patients are screened for medical necessity as health insurance companies will not provide coverage for health-related services that do not establish medical necessity (Handlon 2020, 247).

95. c The OIG Work Plan provides insight into what directions CMS will be taking in a given year to combat fraud and abuse; The NCCI is designed to ensure proper CPT and CHPCS coding; the Medicare Claims Processing Manuals delineate day-to-day operating procedures and policies for filing claims as well as statutes and regulations (Casto and White 2021, 200–202).

96. d Each of the three elements of the RBRVS is adjusted to local costs through the GPCIs (Casto and White 2021, 123).

97. d To prove medical necessity, the diagnosis code must be linked to the procedure code. In this case, the procedure code would not be used for selections a, b, or c (Casto and White 2021, 153).

CCS-P MEDICAL SCENARIOS

Exam 4 Scenario 1

DX1	M48.04	Spinal stenosis, thoracic region
DX2	M70.61	Trochanteric bursitis, right hip
DX3	M70.62	Trochanteric bursitis, left hip
DX4	M65.331	Trigger finger, right middle finger
PR1	99214	Office or other outpatient visit for the evaluation and management of an established patient, which requires a medically appropriate history and/or examination and moderate level of medical decision making
PR2	20600	Arthrocentesis, aspiration and/or injection, small joint or bursa (eg, fingers, toes); without ultrasound guidance

PR3	J3301	Injection, triamcinolone acetonide, not otherwise specified, 10 mg
PR4	20610	Arthrocentesis, aspiration and/or injection, major joint or bursa (eg, shoulder, hip, knee, subacromial bursa); without ultrasound guidance
PR5	20610	Arthrocentesis, aspiration and/or injection, major joint or bursa (eg, shoulder, hip, knee, subacromial bursa); without ultrasound guidance

Exam 4 Scenario 2

DX1	K80.50	Calculus of bile duct without cholangitis or cholecystitis without obstruction
PR1	99244	Office consultation for a new or established patient, which requires these 3 key components: a comprehensive history; a comprehensive examination; and medical decision making of moderate complexity

Exam 4 Scenario 3

DX1	I65.21	Occlusion and stenosis of right carotid artery
PR1	35301	Thromboendarterectomy, including patch graft, if performed; carotid, vertebral, subclavian, by neck incision

Exam 4 Scenario 4

DX1	H05.112	Granuloma of left orbit
PR1	68510	Biopsy of lacrimal gland

Exam 4 Scenario 5

DX1	K52.9	Noninfective gastroenteritis and colitis, unspecified
DX2	E86.0	Dehydration
PR1	96360	Intravenous infusion, hydration; initial, 31 minutes to 1 hour

Exam 4 Scenario 6

DX1	Z23	Encounter for immunization
PR1	90700	Diphtheria, tetanus toxoids, and acellular pertussis vaccine (DTaP), when administered to individuals younger than 7 years, for intramuscular use
PR2	90460	Immunization administration through 18 years of age via any route of administration, with counseling by physician or other qualified health care professional first or only component of each vaccine or toxoid administered
PR3	90461	each additional vaccine or toxoid component administered (List separately in addition to code for primary procedure)
PR4	90461	each additional vaccine or toxoid component administered (List separately in addition to code for primary procedure)

Exam 4 Scenario 7

DX1	J44.1	Chronic obstructive pulmonary disease with (acute) exacerbation
DX2	C91.11	Chronic lymphocytic leukemia of B-cell type in remission
PR1	99214	Office or other outpatient visit for the evaluation and management of an established patient, which requires a medically appropriate history and/or examination and moderate level of medical decision making

Exam 4 Scenario 8

DX1	T86.11	Kidney transplant rejection
DX2	N18.6	End stage renal disease
DX3	T86.12	Kidney transplant failure
PR1	50370	Removal of transplanted renal allograft

REFERENCES

The following resources are referenced in the Answer Key:

ACDIS-AHIMA. 2019 (February). Practice Brief: Guidelines for Achieving a Complaint Query Practice. https://acdis.org/resources/guidelines-achieving-compliant-query-practice%E2%80%942019-update.

American Medical Association. 2022. *CPT Professional Edition 2022*. Chicago: AMA.

American Medical Association. 2012. *CPT Changes 2012: An Insider's View*. Chicago: AMA.

American Medical Association. *CPT Assistant*, 1990 through 2018 editions. Chicago: AMA.

Bowman, S. 2017. Corporate Compliance. Chapter 18 in *Fundamentals of Law for Health Informatics and Information Management,* 3rd ed. Edited by M. Brodnik, L. Rinehart-Thompson, and R. Reynolds. Chicago: AHIMA.

Brinda, D. and A. Watters. 2020. Data Privacy, Confidentiality, and Security. Chapter 11 in *Health Information Management: Concepts, Principles, and Practice*, 6th ed. Edited by P. Oachs and A. Watters. Chicago: AHIMA.

Casto, A. B. and S. White. 2021. *Principles of Healthcare Reimbursement*, 7th ed. Chicago: AHIMA.

Centers for Disease Control and Prevention, Centers for Medicare and Medicaid Services and the National Center for Health Statistics. 2021. *ICD-10-CM Official Guidelines for Coding and Reporting 2022*. https://www.cms.gov/files/document/fy-2022-icd-10-cm-coding-guidelines -updated-02012022.pdf.

Centers for Medicare and Medicaid Services (CMS). 2022. HCPCS Quarterly Update. https://www.cms .gov/Medicare/Coding/HCPCSReleaseCodeSets/HCPCS-Quarterly-Update.

Centers for Medicare and Medicaid Services (CMS). 2021a. Medicare Claims Processing Manual. Chapter 12, Sections 30.6.9 & 30.6.12 (A–J): 54–56. https://www.cms.gov/Regulations-and -Guidance/Guidance/Manuals/downloads/clm104c01.pdf.

Centers for Medicare and Medicaid Services (CMS). 2021b. National Correct Coding Initiative Edits. https://www.cms.gov/Medicare/Coding/NationalCorrectCodInitEd.

Central Office on ICD-10-CM/PCS. 2021. *AHA Coding Clinic for ICD-10-CM and ICD-10-PCS*. Third Quarter.

Central Office on ICD-10-CM/PCS. 2021. *AHA Coding Clinic for ICD-10-CM and ICD-10-PCS*. Fourth Quarter.

Handlon, L. 2020. Revenue Cycle Management. Chapter 8 in *Health Information Management: Concepts, Principles, and Practice,* 6th ed. Edited by P. Oachs and A. Watters. Chicago: AHIMA.

Hazelwood, A. and C. Venable. 2014. *Diagnostic Coding for Physician Services*. Chicago: AHIMA.

Huey, K. 2021. *Procedural Coding and Reimbursement for Physician Services: Applying Current Procedural Terminology and HCPCS*. Chicago: AHIMA.

Hunt, T. J. and K. Kirk. 2020. Clinical Documentation Improvement and Coding Compliance. Chapter 9 in *Health Information Management: Concepts, Principles, and Practice*, 6th ed. Edited by P. Oachs and A. Watters. Chicago: AHIMA.

Klaver, J. 2017. Consent to Treatment. Chapter 8 in *Fundamentals of Law for Health Informatics and Information Management,* 3rd ed. Edited by M. Brodnik, L. Rinehart-Thompson, and R. Reynolds. Chicago: AHIMA.

LeBlanc, M. M. 2020. Human Resources Management. Chapter 22 in *Health Information Management: Concepts, Principles, and Practice,* 6th ed. Edited by P. Oachs and A. Watters. Chicago: AHIMA.

Leon-Chisen, N. 2022. *ICD-10-CM and ICD-10-PCS Coding Handbook 2022 with Answers*. Chicago: American Hospital Association.

Mosby's Medical Dictionary, 10th ed. 2017. St. Louis, MO: Elsevier.

Olenik, K. and R. Reynolds. 2017. Security Threats and Controls. Chapter 13 in *Fundamentals of Law for Health Informatics and Information Management,* 3rd ed. Edited by M. Brodnik, L. Rinehart-Thompson, and R. Reynolds. Chicago: AHIMA.

Optum360. 2022. *ICD-10-CM Expert for Hospitals*: *The Complete Official Code Set*. Salt Lake City: Optum360.

Prescribers' Digital Reference (PDR). 2021. Depo-Provera Sterile Aqueous Suspension (Medroxyprogesterone Acetate). http://www.pdr.net/drug-summary/Depo-Provera-Sterile -Aqueous-Suspension-medroxyprogesterone-acetate-2875.8223.

Prescribers' Digital Reference (PDR). 2022a. Levothyroxine sodium. https://www.pdr.net/drug -summary/Synthroid-levothyroxine-sodium-26.643.

Prescribers' Digital Reference (PDR). 2022b. Haloperidol. https://www.pdr.net/drug-summary /Haldol-haloperidol-942.

Reynolds, R. and A. Morey. 2020. Health Record Content and Documentation. Chapter 4 in *Health Information Management: Concepts, Principles, and Practice*, 6th ed. Edited by P. Oachs and A. Watters. Chicago: AHIMA.

Reynolds, R. and M. Brodnik. 2017. The HIPAA Security Rule. Chapter 12 in *Fundamentals of Law for Health Informatics and Information Management,* 3rd ed. Edited by M. Brodnik, L. Rinehart-Thompson, and R. Reynolds. Chicago: AHIMA.

Rinehart-Thompson, L. 2017a. HIPAA Privacy Rule: Part I. Chapter 10 in *Fundamentals of Law for Health Informatics and Information Management,* 3rd ed. Edited by M. Brodnik, L. Rinehart-Thompson, and R. Reynolds. Chicago: AHIMA.

Rinehart-Thompson, L. 2017b. HIPAA Privacy Rule: Part II. Chapter 11 in *Fundamentals of Law for Health Informatics and Information Management,* 3rd ed. Edited by M. Brodnik, L. Rinehart-Thompson, and R. Reynolds. Chicago: AHIMA.

Schraffenberger, L. A. and B. Palkie. 2022. *Basic ICD-10-CM and ICD-10-PCS Coding,* 2022. Chicago: AHIMA.

Smith, G. I. 2021. *Basic Current Procedural Terminology and HCPCS Coding*. Chicago: AHIMA.

Watson, M. 2018 (June). Documentation and Coding Practices for Risk Adjustment and Hierarchical Condition Categories. *Journal of AHIMA* 89(6).

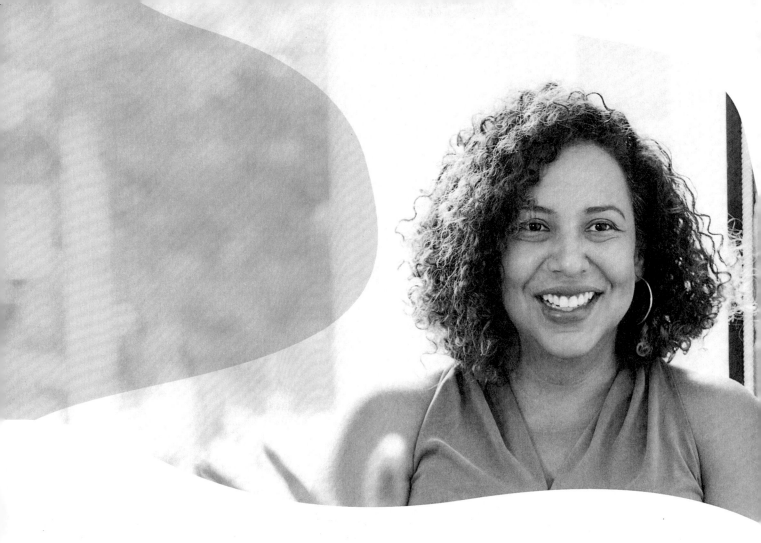

Discover, Connect, Advance

Join AHIMA, and join a community of passionate, forward-thinking health information professionals driving progress in the world of healthcare.

Find success as an AHIMA member though:

- Discounts in the AHIMA Store on education and certification resources
- More than 50 percent off Continuing Education maintenance
- Complimentary Continuing Education Units
- Timely articles weekly through the Journal of AHIMA and the E-Alert weekly newsletter
- Early notification about new jobs posted on the Career Assist: Job Bank site
- Networking opportunities at the state and national level
- Our members-only social platform, access, discuss hot topics, talk with and learn from other members, and explore and share AHIMA educationand news
- Tools to affect health information public policy

Join today at ahima.org/join

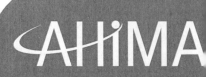